OPEN
LIVES
Safe Schools

edited by
Donovan R. Walling

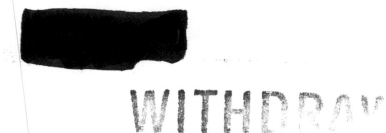
WITHDRAW

Phi Delta Kappa Educational Foundation
Bloomington, Indiana

Cover design by
Victoria Voelker

Library of Congress Catalog Card Number 95-71812
ISBN 0-87367-485-5
Copyright © 1996 by Phi Delta Kappa Educational Foundation
Bloomington, Indiana

Table of Contents

Part Three: Youth, Parents, and Families

Part Four: Responses

Part Five: Resources

Introduction

In all but a handful of states (only nine at the time this book went to press), it is legal to discriminate against an individual on the basis of sexual orientation. Landlords can — and often do — refuse to rent to gay or lesbian individuals or couples. Businesses can refuse to hire gay workers or can fire a worker solely — and openly — because that worker is (or is suspected of being) gay or lesbian.

At the federal level, military service still is open only to gay and lesbian members who stay "in the closet" under the "don't ask, don't tell" policy compromise worked out by the Clinton Administration and a homophobic military establishment. Only a few states, some municipalities in other states, and some businesses and school districts include sexual orientation among the characteristics, such as race, religion, and ethnicity, that define their nondiscrimination statutes and policies.

Thus it is little wonder that most schools are affected by anti-gay discrimination. Few schools can — or choose to — challenge their state's or community's prejudices to address the needs of gay and lesbian students, parents, teachers, administrators, and staff. And, absent nondiscrimination protection, education professionals often are reluctant to deal with gay and lesbian issues that affect themselves and their students for fear that they, too, will fall victim to open, sanctioned discrimination.

Open Lives, Safe Schools is written for all educators and other readers concerned about schooling, because homophobia (the unfounded fear of homosexual persons and homosexuality in general) and anti-gay discrimination affect everyone in schools. Anxiety about potential discrimination is as great for many nongay educators as for gay or lesbian educators. Being openly

1

supportive of gay students, gay parents, or gay colleagues can be as professionally (often personally) dangerous as being openly gay or lesbian.

When an individual writes a letter to the editor of a local newspaper and supports gay issues, it is not unusual for the writer to receive harassing and threatening phone calls. One such individual, with whom I am acquainted, awoke one night to find a cross burning on her front lawn. In spite of this incident and repeated telephone harassment, local police turned a blind eye. Even though the harassment was clearly illegal, anti-gay discrimination in that location is not. Under similar circumstances in other places, discrimination often is blatant; and hurtful, illegal actions, such as telephone harassment and cross-burnings that are motivated by anti-gay prejudice, frequently are treated lightly, if at all.

More than any other political movement in recent memory, the so-called Religious Right has spread a systematic campaign of hatred and intolerance that targets gay men and lesbians for harassment and discrimination. An avowed goal of the Religious Right is to take over America's schools in order to impose their values on all children and educators. The Religious Right's "fundamentalist" rantings are thin cover for a pervasive power lust. Unfortunately, many religious fundamentalists who are honestly concerned about their children's education have been swept into the Religious Right's political tide. Thus cloaked in religiosity, those who would abuse and harass homosexuals do so with relative impunity.

Senator Jesse Helms (R-N.C.), the Religious Right's primary congressional ally, frequently offers examples of outright discrimination. Not long ago, in the congressional debate over the reauthorization of the Elementary and Secondary Education Act, Senator Helms was instrumental in putting forward an amendment in the form of a social-issue rider that would have prevented ESEA dollars from being used "to carry out a program or activity that has either the purpose or effect of encouraging or supporting homosexuality as a positive lifestyle alternative." Senate-House conferees reached a compromise that blunted this flagrantly discriminatory rider, settling eventually on language that prohibits schools from using ESEA funds to "promote or encourage sexual activity, whether heterosexual or homosexual."[1]

Representative Steve Gunderson (R-Wis.), one of the conferees and an openly gay congressman, helped to frame the compromise, but not before being heatedly challenged on a personal level regarding his own sexual orientation by Representative Robert Dornan (R-Calif.).

Had the Helms amendment become part of the reauthorization of ESEA, educators could have been prevented from giving students information about sexual orientation issues or telling questioning students about such resources as books, educational videos, support groups, and telephone hotlines. The result would have been, in effect, to censor legitimate educational dialogue. As educators' self-censorship already denies many students information that they need to make informed decisions about their lives, such formalized prior restraint would have put more students at risk.

The central premise of *Open Lives, Safe Schools* is that allowing students, parents, educators, and others who are part of the school community — from kindergarten through graduate school — to live openly in terms of sexual orientation is healthy for everyone. The authors of these essays address a number of important gay and lesbian issues in education, from the coming-out processes of students and adults to gay-positive/gay-visible curricula to parenting and family concerns.

The essays are grouped into five sections. Part I addresses professional issues, starting with Jan Goodman's personal view and including the first-person accounts of John D. Anderson, Tony Prince, and Dan Woog.

Part II moves on to curricular issues. The section opens with Arthur Lipkin's foundational piece, "The Case for a Gay and Lesbian Curriculum." John Warren Stewig and Vicky Greenbaum look at literature issues in elementary and secondary classrooms. Then, in essays from geographically diverse settings, three authors examine gay and lesbian studies in higher education. Alan Sinfield provides a view from the United Kingdom, David Phillips from Australia, and Henry Gonshak from the American West. Finally, Ian Barnard offers a checklist of suggestions for teachers who wish to counter homophobic attitudes.

Part III focuses on youth, parents, and families. The section begins with the coming-out story from Lynn Johnston's popular newspaper comic strip, "For Better or For Worse." David Aveline and Kathryn Brown's insightful study of questions received by college student panels on gay and lesbian issues is next, followed by Jill Gover's perspective on "Gay Youth in the Family." High school student Shulamit Kleinerman provides a student viewpoint in her essay, "Old Enough to Know." The last essay in this section is James Sears' comprehensive treatment, "Challenges for Educators: Lesbian, Gay, and Bisexual Families."

Part IV concentrates on individual, school, and community responses to gay and lesbian issues. Rita Kissen's compelling account of the effects of anti-gay ballot initiatives in Colorado and Oregon sets the stage. The next three essays describe effective resource programs: Project 10, IYG, and GLSTN. The article on Project 10 was written by the program's founder, Virginia Uribe. I co-wrote the IYG piece with the gay, lesbian, and bisexual teens support group's founder, the late Christopher Gonzalez, who died just as this book was being developed. Kevin Jennings, yet another pioneer, describes the development of the Gay, Lesbian, and Straight Teachers Network. Finally, Frances Snowder examines gay teen suicide and ways to prevent it.

Part V is a collection of resources, which is divided into sections for 1) bibliographies, resource guides, and directories; 2) curricula and professional issues; 3) parents and families; 4) periodicals; 5) youth groups; and 6) youth issues. Included are both print and nonprint resources and important names and addresses of key organizations.

At a fundamental level, schools will not be safe places for gay and lesbian individuals — and, by association, for others in schools — until being gay or lesbian is destigmatized. Schools cannot be safe until being honest and open about one's sexuality is valued and affirmed at every level.

The risks of growing up gay and lesbian are real and, for sensitive educators and parents, all too familiar. Students who are confused about their sexual orientation or feel despondent or rejected because of their homosexuality are at risk of school failure, at the very least, when such feelings interfere with their studies. Those whose despondency or isolation is unrelieved risk worse fates. The suicide rate for gay and lesbian teens is three times that of heterosexual teens. And those whose confusion is left to be resolved not by communication, but through sexual trial and error, risk contracting sexually transmitted diseases, including AIDS. The statistics on teenage AIDS incidence are alarming. Not long ago, a report concluded that one in four persons with AIDS in Georgia is a teenager; in Los Angeles and Miami, 20% of reported AIDS cases are teens; in Newark, New Jersey, the figure is 35%.[2]

In an earlier publication I stated that:

> Fear of controversy, cultural taboos, and to some degree, an irrational fear of homosexuality have prevented many educators from dealing effectively with gay and lesbian young people. . . . The climate in most schools is such that gay teens rarely are willing to expose themselves to the ridicule, harassment, and abuse that comes when they openly acknowledge their sexual orientation. . . . To counteract these conditions, educators will need to acknowledge that homosexuality is a variation in sexual orientation and that they have a professional responsibility to provide information, counseling, and other services to help gay teens understand their sexual orientation and to avoid high-risk behaviors. They will need to regard homophobic prejudice in the same light as other prejudices, such as racism or anti-Semitism. And they will need to take deliberate steps to eliminate the negative attitudes and actions of students and staff in their schools that place gay teens at risk.[3]

All of this is equally true for gay and lesbian adults in schools. Jan Goodman, in her essay in this book, "Lesbian, Gay, and Bisexual Issues in Education: A Personal View," writes:

> Lesbian, gay, and bisexual staff members are often alone in the fight against homophobia. Often, we feel we have the most to lose by confronting it. We are told that the issue is not important, or that it is solely our issue, or that there is no issue to be dealt with at all. At the same time, religious fundamentalists launch countless initiatives in attempts to deny us the right to be ourselves or to outlaw any mention of homosexuality in the curriculum. We desperately need heterosexual allies to join us as leaders in this fight, with voices that can be heard, and the power to affect change.

Increasingly, the Religious Right is influencing the political process and affecting the ways in which many schools operate and what those schools provide for their students, the students' parents, and school employees in terms of information, support, and safety. Although that movement is not alone in fostering discrimination, it is the most influential. The only way to combat such misinformation and discrimination is by increasing the public's

— and particularly educators' — awareness of gay and lesbian issues that affect schools.

By illuminating and probing these issues, honest dialogue may be generated and real solutions to the problems and concerns that arise from these issues may be found. In the final analysis, the authors of these essays are advocates of safe schools in the most basic sense of safety: Schools should be places where it is safe to be oneself.

Footnotes

1. Mark Pitsch, "In Political Season, 'Social Issue' Add-Ons Bulk Up E.S.E.A.," *Education Week*, 26 October 1994, p. 22.
2. Victoria Brownworth, "America's Worst-Kept Secret," *The Advocate* (March 1992): 38-46.
3. Donovan R. Walling, *Gay Teens at Risk*, Fastback 357 (Bloomington, Ind.: Phi Delta Kappa Educational Foundation, 1993), p. 29.

Part One
Professional Issues

Lesbian, Gay, and Bisexual Issues in Education: A Personal View*

by Jan M. Goodman

Recently, I attended a workshop on diversity at an annual conference for a large educational organization. An administrator from Georgia reported that her school had made great progress in meeting the needs of its increasingly diverse student population, which represented a wide variety of cultures and ethnicities. She proudly told us that the school had bolstered its library collection with books that reflected its students' backgrounds. She also described an International Night, where parents shared food from their homelands. She added that her predominantly white staff had received extensive training on diversity issues.

During the question-and-answer period, I asked, "What are you doing to support the lesbian, gay, and bisexual people in your school community?" She replied, "I doubt that we have any." I informed her that an estimated 10% of the population is gay or lesbian, and that there were likely to be homosexual students, staff, and parents in every school district in the United States. I asked if there were resources in her library that presented a positive view of homosexuality and if her staff's diversity training program included issues of sexual orientation.

*This article first appeared in *Thrust for Educational Leadership* in April 1993. *Thrust* is published by the Association of California School Administrators. Reprinted with permission.

In answering "no," the administrator assured me, again, that there were no gay people in her school community. I responded that no lesbian, gay, or bisexual person would feel comfortable revealing his or her sexual identity in a school atmosphere that denied their existence.

This incident reflects the systematic exclusion of lesbians, gays, and bisexuals that prevails in the large majority of our nation's schools. California is no exception. When dealing with diversity, many of our schools have begun to focus on the needs of groups who have traditionally been denied access and representation in the educational system: people of color, females, and people with disabilities. However, with few exceptions, most school districts fail to acknowledge or serve the needs of lesbian, gay, and bisexual students, parents, and staff.

As a lesbian, I have experienced the pain of exclusion as a student, parent, teacher, and principal in the public school system. I have felt angry, frustrated, and, on rare occasions, hopeful. As an educator, I write this article with the hope that school administrators will have the integrity and the courage to implement policies and practices that are truly inclusive of all members of their community. This may require you to confront and overcome the harmful lessons and false assumptions we have all learned from our homophobic society.

The price of our ignorance can be fatal.

Lesbian, Gay, and Bisexual Students

As a college student in the early 1970s, I recognized my emotional and sexual attraction to women. In vain, I searched for support within the college community. When I looked for books about homosexuality in the university library's card catalogue, I found cross-references to deviance, abnormal psychology, alcoholism, and suicide. There were no books available with positive information about my sexuality.

Alone, isolated and alienated from my family and friends, I asked the counseling center for a therapist who understood and accepted lesbianism. Instead, the center referred me to a therapist who spent four weeks questioning my need to have her "approve" my lifestyle.

Twenty years later, lesbian, gay, and bisexual youth often encounter similar experiences as they come to grips with their sexual orientation in

California's middle and high schools. With little recognition, few resources, and minimal support, they are an at-risk population too often ignored by administrators, teachers, and counselors who are unaware, uninformed, or uncomfortable with same-sex closeness. The price of our ignorance can be fatal.

Lesbian, gay, and bisexual youths face extreme social pressure and commonly feel that in order to "fit in," they must deny their identity. The school curriculum deprives them of lesbian, gay, and bisexual role models who have made contributions to history, mathematics, science, social services, and the arts. They are well aware that they are not welcome to bring same-sex dates to school events and parties.

Students who are openly gay are often the targets of verbal or physical harassment by homophobic peers, and are reluctant to report these incidents for fear of rejection or retribution by classmates, teachers, and counselors. Alienated and depressed, a disproportionate number of lesbian and gay youth have substance abuse problems. Many run away from home; others attempt suicide. Sadly, some succeed.

Lesbian, Gay, and Bisexual Parents and Families

For five years, I lived with my lover and two children. The four of us were clearly a family, and I was involved in every aspect of their daily lives. Yet when we registered the boys for elementary school and junior high, there was no place for me on the enrollment form or emergency card. The school ignored my existence until our son ran into some typically adolescent trouble in school. Then, school officials did not hesitate to state that he had gotten in with a "bad crowd" because of our "abnormal lifestyle." Needless to say, they did not blame the poor behavior of his co-conspirators on the fact that they all had heterosexual parents!

When we enroll our children in school, lesbian, gay, and bisexual parents — as well as other non-traditional families — fight for legitimization. In elementary school, students routinely are asked to make Mother's Day and Father's Day cards, whether or not they have a mom or a dad, or whether they have two moms, two dads, or an extended family of grandparents, aunts, uncles, and friends.

Often, parents are hesitant to reveal their homosexuality to another parent, teacher, or principal for fear of judgments, false child-abuse accusations, or — at worst — losing custody of their children. Co-parents are not usually considered "authentic" sources of information about a student. Rarely is a parent's same-sex partner invited to a conference, a PTA meeting, or a field trip.

Children of same-sex parents receive a mixed message. At home, their family is a natural, acceptable, and loving unit. Yet when they arrive at most schools, they see only heterosexual families validated in the stories that they read or in the assumptions made by their teachers.

Schools are often the first place children from lesbian and gay families learn the insults that describe their mothers or fathers. They learn that one of the worst accusations someone can make about you is to say you're gay. They see boys fight to defend their masculinity when classmates taunt them with the word "fag." They are torn between positive and negative images about their family and realize that it may not be safe to defend those they love. In fact, some children may feel they need to join in the verbal gay bashing so no one will suspect their family is not "normal." Too often, homophobic behavior is ignored by teachers and principals. At best, we tell students they should not make hurtful comments to other people. We assure the victims that words can never harm them. We deal with the symptom, but we rarely confront the underlying assumption that being gay or lesbian is an insult to someone. By failing to confront homophobic attitudes in students, schools become agents of injustice.

Lesbian, Gay, and Bisexual Staff Members

For 12 years, I taught grades K-5 in urban schools with diverse populations. At first, I avoided all pronouns when discussing my private life. Even after I told the staff I was a lesbian, I was faced with assumptions that I was heterosexual, or that my lesbianism was simply a stage of life that I would soon outgrow.

After I brought my lover to a social event, a colleague insensitively offered to introduce me to her male cousin. In the staff room one morning, I was shocked when I complained about an upset stomach and a teacher assumed that my birth control method had failed and I was pregnant.

As an elementary school principal in Newark, Calif., my life was compartmentalized. Each day, as I entered the school building, I hung my jacket and an important part of myself in the closet. I then spent the day building self-esteem in my students, while painfully chipping away at my own. While I stayed in the closet, the school community in my district missed out on an important lesson about respect and justice for all.

Although California has recently enacted a law that prohibits employment discrimination based on sexual orientation, many teachers and administrators feel hesitant to tell the whole truth about our lives. Too many of us still fear we will lose our jobs or be labeled incompetent under the guise of effective supervision. Some of us feel we have to be twice as effective as our heterosexual colleagues because of this increased job risk.

Schools are often the first place children from lesbian and gay families learn the insults that describe their mothers or fathers.

Our behavior is labeled inappropriate if we dare to "come out" to our students and provide role models for the 10% who will be lesbian or gay, or the 90% who need to know and respect homosexuals so that they can expand their view of the world. We are accused of causing trouble, or proselytizing our lifestyle with the intent to "convert" others.

Administrators may closely monitor teachers who are openly lesbian, gay, or bisexual to be sure that we do not overstep our bounds with students, regardless of the fact that almost all reported incidents of sexual harassment of students have been perpetrated by heterosexual males. When we are true to ourselves in the school setting, we risk becoming targets of false rumors, verbal harassment, and unsubstantiated child-abuse charges. These attitudes and assumptions cause undue stress to competent teachers and administrators.

Lesbian, gay, and bisexual staff members are often alone in the fight against homophobia. Often, we feel we have the most to lose by confronting it. We are told that the issue is not important, or that it is solely our issue, or that there is no issue to be dealt with at all. At the same time, religious fundamentalists launch countless initiatives in attempts to deny us the right to be ourselves or to outlaw any mention of homosexuality in the curriculum. We desperately need heterosexual allies to join us as leaders in this fight, with voices that can be heard, and the power to affect change.

Assumptions and Excuses

Why is it that many schools are reluctant to adopt policies and practices that prohibit discrimination on the basis of sexual orientation and include lesbians, gay men, and bisexuals as part of the curriculum and social structure? In 20 years as an educator, I continue to hear many false assumptions about homosexuality. I present and respond to them with the hope that school administrators will understand that these assumptions are merely excuses to deny human rights to one-tenth of our school community. When the assumptions are given credence in schools, they are obstacles to change.

ASSUMPTION: There are no gay people in my school. Everyone is or will grow up to be heterosexual.

REALITY: If you create an atmosphere in which every person feels safe to be herself, you will discover that there are lesbian, gay, and bisexual students, parents, and staff in every school district.

ASSUMPTION: My students are too young to learn about sex. They won't understand.

REALITY: When you teach children that there are many ways to live and to be happy, they are learning about diversity, tolerance, and respect for differences.

ASSUMPTION: We've made great progress dealing with racism and sexism in our school. Isn't that enough?

REALITY: It is not enough. No school environment is safe until it is free of all forms of discrimination.

ASSUMPTION: This issue is too controversial. I don't want to alienate anyone.

REALITY: Human rights issues are always controversial. That is because our society thrives on a system in which some people must be "better" than others.

ASSUMPTION: Teaching about homosexuality will cause such a stir that it will interfere with the educational process.

No school environment is safe until it is free of all forms of discrimination.

14

REALITY: Teaching about respect is fundamental to the educational process.

ASSUMPTION: This is a moral issue. Schools should not teach morality.

REALITY: It is a moral issue when an at-risk population is systematically excluded from representation and resources in the educational system.

ASSUMPTION: If students have lesbian/gay/bisexual teachers as role models, they will be "recruited" to become homosexual.

REALITY: Our goal is to educate students. Like all under-represented groups, lesbian, gay, and bisexual students need adult role models so that they will feel more comfortable with who they are. We can't "cause" homosexuality, but we can prevent suicide.

ASSUMPTION: Homosexuality is not normal and not natural. How can I pretend that I accept it?

REALITY: It is unacceptable to deny human rights because of a personal prejudice or belief. If we are to be responsible leaders in the educational community, these attitudes must be set aside or overcome in order to ensure equity for all students.

ASSUMPTION: I agree that this issue is important, but it's so overwhelming that I don't know where to begin.

REALITY: There are a number of successful models and resources available to help schools deal with diversity in terms of sexual orientation. As a first step, duplicate this article for your entire staff. Then, use it as a springboard for discussion and a basis to begin a close examination of whether your school climate supports all students, parents, and staff.

Conclusion

In summary, the school community is a microcosm of the entire society. We are charged with the implementation of our country's goals for the future. We mirror our society's values and, too often, its prejudices. As architects of change, our goal must be to create a blueprint of policies and practices to ensure that each member of our school community is validated and respected. Anything short of this goal is a travesty.

Out as a Professional Educator

by John D. Anderson

For centuries, an "out" educator was practically an oxymoron. Certainly in this country, the last place the ill-informed or religiously biased have wanted gays or lesbians has been in the position of role models for children. Nevertheless, as in every profession, gays and lesbians are working in education. They are at every level, from teachers in the classroom to the highest administrative positions. And, of course, this includes the board of education. But only in the last few years have gay and lesbian educators been "coming out."

"Coming out" is an ambiguous expression with multiple meanings. Clearly, it conveys a process, not an event. However, coming out for an educator entails a variety of phases and, most important, a variety of audiences. Revealing one's homosexuality to a professional colleague is miles apart from revealing one's sexual orientation to students. Yet both are happening and both are necessary.

In September 1991, when I came out to my school system, colleagues, students, and parents, I wanted to do so in order to help our hiding, hurting gay and lesbian students. This seemed necessity enough. However, as the months rolled by and the conversation on diversity and equity evolved, I found a different, additional necessity: to combat the culture of homophobia rampant and essentially unchallenged in our schools.

Lately, I have seen yet another reason for coming out. We are educating the entire student population partly for success in the workplace. We do them a disservice if we fail to bring them face to face with their own prejudices or fail to facilitate their thinking about them now. Our students will enter a world of work where they will work for, over, and beside gay and lesbian colleagues. If they do not understand their own prejudices and lack experience in dealing productively with those prejudices, they may be in danger of losing their jobs.

Nine states already punish anti-gay/lesbian discrimination in the workplace. Eventually, there will be more. In addition, in 1994 the Employment Non-Discrimination Act (ENDA) was introduced in both houses of Congress with a record number of sponsors. It is possible that before too long federal legislation may exist to protect all gay and lesbian citizens in the workplace.

Preliminary Considerations

In addressing issues of coming out or being out in an education setting, there are several considerations to be taken into account. Foremost is the pioneering aspect of this entire effort. Before 1984, there was no Project 10. Before 1985, there was no Harvey Milk High School in New York City. Before 1988, the National Education Association was silent on issues of sexual orientation. Before 1993, not even one state had passed a law protecting gay students from discrimination. As recently as May 1994, *Educational Leadership* published a dozen articles around the theme, "Education for Diversity," with nary a mention of gays or lesbians.

Agents of change always face difficulties. Agents of change on the issue of equitable education for gays and lesbians face a particularly harrowing challenge, which brings us to another important consideration.

The entire effort to achieve equity on issues of sexual orientation rings hollow without openly gay and lesbian participants. Heterosexuals cannot do it for us. We must be there on the front lines. Students, whether gay or straight, mock our efforts when they can ask, "If being gay is okay, where are all the gay and lesbian teachers?" Role models must come forward if there is to be progress. However, this is not a condemnation of closeted gays and lesbians. Coming out is no exception to the ancient wisdom, "To everything there is a season."

Concomitant with this latter aspect of the issue are two further considerations. First, people contribute in a myriad of ways. The health teacher may be hiding; but if he or she invites openly gay or lesbian speakers to address the class, this teacher is making a valuable contribution. A supervisor may be closeted; but if he or she suggests strategies that permit or invite openness on a broader level, then this educator also is making a positive contribution. Allies come in varied shapes and sizes.

Second, gay and lesbian educators cannot do it all by themselves. They must learn to trust their heterosexual colleagues. Schools are filled with hetero-heroes, who see the need but don't know how to address it. When they look for leadership, too often the potential leaders are silent.

The Stratford Model

How awareness of the needs of gay and lesbian students and educators emerged in the public schools of Stratford, Connecticut, illustrates these points.

Stratford is a town of about 50,000. To some, it is simply a charming south-shore community; others see it as a too-close suburb of a blighted city, Bridgeport. Actually, Stratford is both.

The school system comprises two high schools, two middle schools, and nine elementary schools. I began teaching in Stratford in 1985, my fourth year in the profession.

In 1991, three events converged to change my life as a teacher. First, in October, Connecticut's law to extend civil rights protection to gay and lesbian citizens went into effect. Second, during the late summer of that year, I was selected by the *New Haven Register* to take over the writing of a bimonthly column on gay and lesbian issues. Third, for my official evaluation goal for the 1991-92 school year, I chose to examine the needs of gay and lesbian students and to evaluate how the school system was meeting those needs.

The passage of protective legislation encouraged me to step into a position that I had hardly imagined possible: writing an opinion column on gay and lesbian issues for a major Connecticut urban daily. Similarly, the new law provided a sufficiently protected environment at work to step forward and push the school system to use the "G-word" and the "L-word" for the first

The entire effort to achieve equity on issues of sexual orientation rings hollow without openly gay and lesbian participants.

19

time. In spite of this legislated level of comfort, both decisions took a good deal of soul-searching.

Would either of these actions have taken place without the supportive legal environment? I like to think they would have. However, I am sure progress would have been slower, because opposition would have been stronger. Or, at least, cooperation from colleagues would have been more limited and tentative. A politically active co-worker told me that my efforts were discussed at a meeting of the Republican Town Committee. One man was heard to say, "We've got to put an end to Anderson's activities." Eyebrows were raised, but an awareness of state law put an end to the discussion. Nothing came of it.

A global sort of ignorance arises from the fact that homosexuals have been the focus of prejudice and misconceptions for centuries.

The Connecticut law has created an environment conducive to progress on sexual orientation issues much as capitalism and the free enterprise system create an environment for the business community. What has happened throughout the state is directly attributable to individual courage, ingenuity, and creativity, to be sure. However, every step has been bolstered by an atmosphere of legal near-equality.

During my first year as an out educator, I came to realize that many initiatives on the issue of equity education for gay and lesbian students had already begun. There was a clear professional mandate to strive for a safe and equitable school environment for gay and lesbian students and staff. The National Education Association and the American Federation of Teachers, as well as the Connecticut Education Association, all had passed resolutions of support. What stood in the way of implementing any of these resolutions was ignorance and a lack of leadership.

For one thing, hardly anyone was aware of the stand of the education profession on the issue. Not until 1992 did the Connecticut State Department of Education, through its *Sex Equity Newsletter,* address homophobia and suggest ways to create more equitable schools for gay and lesbian people. This was done with a single-page entry in the newsletter. And the newsletter piece was clearly the work of the Sex Equity Consultant, not a department policy statement.

During 1993, a small group of gay and lesbian educators and friends of education started meeting to plan a statewide teachers' group. The result of these meetings has been the formation of the fledgling EdFLAG (Educators and Friends of Lesbians and Gays). The organization provides a network, informative workshops and speakers, and a sense of community for professionals grappling with questions of equity in schools.

During 1994-95, the Graduate School of Social Work of the University of Connecticut sponsored a highly successful conference titled, "Children of the Shadows." Workshops and speakers addressed the needs of gay, lesbian, and bisexual students. A few schools, both private and public, have formed student Gay-Straight Alliances. Countless presentations have been made, mostly for the professional staff. The Connecticut Education Association's professional development specialist, Margaret Mahland, sent a letter to every district superintendent offering a workshop on gay and lesbian issues. In fact, she was one of the first people I contacted when I began my journey as an out educator. Her advice was valuable; her assistance has been constant.

A global sort of ignorance arises from the fact that homosexuals have been the focus of prejudice and misconceptions for centuries. Public condemnation from pillar to pulpit have been mirrored in more personal ways in disapproval and rejection by friends and family. Most gay and lesbian people have internalized this intense animosity to at least some extent. Some have allowed it to cripple them and keep them deep in the closet. But Connecticut's progress of the past few years has made a difference in Stratford.

The school board and administration in Stratford have moved slowly from a state of paralysis to one of tentative support for gay and lesbian issues on a case-by-case basis. Incidents of homophobia are dealt with as unacceptable incidents of bias, as they should be. The conversation on gay concerns has progressed and broadened. However, support remains sporadic and unpredictable. There are still pockets of opposition and intransigence. For example, it took two years of lobbying and the threat of a lawsuit to get the school system to grant permission for me to address a senior health class. They did so under pressure from the Stratford Education Association's counsel. Ironically, this incident occurred after the administration had granted me a paid professional day to make a similar presentation at a public high school in nearby West Hartford.

A second example: A questionnaire on homophobia for teachers and administrators that had been developed by a professor of education at nearby Fairfield University was administered at one high school without incident. But the survey was banned from the other high school.

In another instance, a *New York Times* article about me and my efforts on behalf of gay and lesbian students was denied inclusion in a library display titled, "People at Stratford High School We're Proud Of." In a supportive move, the same article was posted on at least two classroom bulletin boards in the high school at the initiative of individual teachers.

As time has passed and positive information about gay men and lesbians has increasingly appeared in the press, progress has been made. A contribution to this positive information, for Stratford, has been my regular column in the *New Haven Register*. (New Haven is only a 20-minute drive from Stratford.) Several of my colleagues have commented positively to me about these columns. This forum for philosophy, views, and opinions has helped to enlarge the general conversation about gay and lesbian issues.

Testing the Waters for Coming Out

Another important impetus for progress has come from a different phenomenon in Stratford. The Stratford public schools now have an openly gay high school teacher, an openly gay elementary school principal (my partner, Garrett), an openly gay middle school teacher, and a middle school assistant principal who is very open about one of her sons being gay. Other gay and lesbian staff members who still are closeted hold district-level administrative positions and teaching positions at both high schools, both middle schools, and at least several elementary schools. There is no formal organization or network for them, but each in his or her own way has been strengthened by the events and progress of the last few years.

My own testing of the waters and the clear staff support that I have received encouraged these staff members to come out. Nothing was planned. Nothing was coordinated. But support definitely has flowed from each of us to the others. We have spoken countless times in person or by phone. Garrett and I have brainstormed our moves. We were there to give support to the somewhat troubled mother when her son came out to her two years ago.

All three of us have experienced moments of fear. Each of us has paid an emotional price for our honesty. Nevertheless, none of us has regrets. The three of us were there for the middle school teacher who was outed by his students. His coming out at work was not a choice. He suffered verbal abuse as only seventh- and eighth-graders can give. But a year later he reported to me a conversation by two of his students.

Student A: Mr. B, you sure look awful today.
Student B: Mr. B has been rehearsing every night this week. He's in the Gay Men's Chorus. Leave him alone. He's tired.

Now, that's progress!

By and large, our colleagues' reactions have been overwhelmingly supportive. Once people have worked with colleagues, the added awareness of their differing sexual orientations takes on less importance. A relationship of respect already has been formed. New information is assimilated and rarely jars the relationship to any significant degree.

The Stratford Education Association was supportive from day one. I spoke to SEA representatives when administration static over my choice of an evaluation goal arose in September 1991. The concern of the SEA centered not on me, but on possible repercussions for Garrett, who was then in his first year as an elementary principal. I assured them that Garrett and I had weighed various aspects of the issue. Finally, I asked them what the SEA would do if Garrett received negative parent reactions. They responded, "Circle the wagons."

I knew I was in good hands. At the end of the 1991-92 school year, at the SEA dinner to honor retirees and others, I was given a Human Affairs Award for my efforts on behalf of gay and lesbian students.

. . . people who know or work with gay or lesbian people have less of a problem with their differences.

Student Reactions

Student reaction has come on three levels. The students in my own classes have been very supportive. They have made comments to me privately and even given me letters of encouragement. When one of them slips and uses "faggot" in a conversation within my hearing, the others giggle and look at me, waiting for my response. I intervene gently and suggest the student use a different word. I point out the similarity to saying "nigger." I try to keep it light, never stripping the student of his dignity. My comments are brief, to the point, and then we move on to something else.

A second level of student reaction has come in the halls of the high school where I teach. Some time ago, on two separate occasions, comments were directed to me about being a "faggot." Both times I took the situation to the principal, who spoke to the students and even required them to apologize to me.

The third level of student response came from outside Stratford, when the student editor of the high school newspaper in the nearby town where I live asked me to write a piece on homosexuality for that paper. The resulting article prompted two telephoned death threats from high school boys who referred to my article in their school paper. I called the police in both instances. They counseled me to keep a close watch on my house and property and said they would do the same. They also said to take the threats seriously, but to realize that they were probably prank calls, which is exactly what they turned out to be. There were no further occurrences. But as innocuous as these threats were, they took a psychological toll. I felt a sense of personal violation. It took some months to completely recover from the sense of invaded privacy that these calls instilled.

> *. . . gay or lesbian educators need to show their colleagues . . . that it is okay to be gay or lesbian.*

What is instructive in all these student responses is the way in which the level of hostility increased as the students' acquaintance with me decreased. My own students voiced no negative reactions. I am not so naive as to think they harbored none. However, there was sufficient support for me from their peers that even if a student was not thrilled about this gay teacher, he or she said nothing. This is a good start as far as I am concerned. It gave them think time, time to look and listen and see what it meant to be working with a gay teacher.

The students in the hall knew who I was, had probably seen me before, and perhaps had friends in my classes. But the students from the town where I live did not know me at all. I was some stranger who had invaded their comfortable heterosexual world with my homosexual presence by my writing in their school paper. These experiences corroborate the truism that people who know or work with gay or lesbian people have less of a problem with their differences.

Parent responses have been less clear-cut. For the most part, there have been none, at least no negative reactions. If there have been any, they apparently stopped at some level of administration and did not filter down to me or to

24

Garrett at his school. In fact, Garrett enjoys outspoken positive parent support. His PTA is solidly behind him. They like what he does for their kids.

Taking on a New Role

An out educator takes on a new role of consultant, counselor, and advocate. When I started this journey in September 1991, I felt extremely isolated. But as the months went by, I gained a growing feeling of strength. I reached beyond my school district throughout the state for a supportive network. I called everyone I heard of or read about who was involved in diversity issues.

Now, in the past four years I have given more than 30 presentations to education groups (administrators, staff, and students). My efforts have acted as a catalyst to empower others. Teachers have started talking openly about issues of homophobia. They are developing curricula that include the contributions of gay men and lesbians. Staff members also talk more openly about gay and lesbian friends, siblings, and children.

Today, parents of gay and lesbian children also can find someone to talk to. The students themselves can now find guidance personnel who are open to discussing sexual orientation questions and concerns. A student can walk into a guidance office and see a rainbow sticker, a pink triangle, or a bumper sticker that reads, "Homophobia is a Social Disease." These indicators tell the student that it is okay to raise gay and lesbian issues and to ask questions that formerly were taboo.

What is slowly happening is the growth of a school environment where being gay or lesbian is on its way to becoming ordinary. This is at least the case for the adults involved. Garrett has his school's Christmas party at our house. His faculty know me. They interact with us as a couple. There are no secrets or embarrassing silences in our conversations. The once "abominable" has been normalized. This has not happened on its own. It has taken a stretch by all of us, gay and straight.

But while individual bias incidents are handled well, little attempt has been made to educate the student population as a whole on the issue of gay and lesbian inclusion. I sent a note to my principal early in the school year requesting him to address homophobia with the incoming freshmen. In the opening assembly with the ninth-graders, he did indeed include sexual orientation in his comments about mutual respect. This same administrator followed up when a ninth-grade student announced in one of my classes, "I want to get out of this class. I want to be around straight people." The principal spoke to the student, probed his reasons for the comment, acknowledged that I was gay, and told him his comment was totally unacceptable.

But Stratford also has a long way to go toward full affirmation. In my school, posters displaying gay and lesbian information are not allowed in the halls. National Gay and Lesbian History Month (October) and Gay and Lesbian Book Month (June) go unacknowledged. There has been no attempt, as yet, by the systemwide curriculum committee to formulate a policy of inclusion. There are no ongoing professional development programs offered to teachers on gay and lesbian issues. For example, some of us have suggested that the B'nai Brith's "World of Difference" diversity training presenters be required to broaden their concept of diversity to include gay and lesbian issues. Although this training program, routinely used by the district, deals exclusively with issues of bias against Jews and Blacks in its manuals and literature, it does provide a general heightened sensitivity to diversity.

Gay and lesbian speakers are brought in to health classes only when individual teachers make this happen. And the administration's health coordinator sits silent on the issue. The language arts supervisor gets excited about inclusion when it means Pacific Rim, African-American, or Holocaust literature. He has adamantly refused to include gay- and lesbian-positive materials.

Conclusion

Coming out as an educator has been a sometimes exhausting, sometimes frightening, sometimes exhilarating experience. It affects every level of a person's being. Every human interaction is awash with honesty and the real possibility for growth, productivity, and satisfaction. Common sense, reflection, and humor are absolute necessities. Patience is required, too.

From attending a few PFLAG meetings and listening to parents, I have learned an important truth. When a child comes out to his or her parents, the child must give the parents time to get used to the new reality. What the child has agonized over and perhaps lived with for months or years, the parents have just learned. The same is true for coming out at work. The gay or lesbian educator usually has lived with the knowledge of his or her sexual orientation for a long time. When they openly acknowledge that sexual orientation, they must give colleagues and students time to process the news. And the newly out educator should not react to every curious look or incautious comment. Those will cease with time.

Professional continuity is a key ingredient in the adjustment of colleagues and students. It is important for out educators to continue to demonstrate by their professional activity that they are the same teachers and administrators their co-workers have always known. Most important, gay or lesbian educators need to show their colleagues, by their own acceptance of who they are, that it is okay to be gay or lesbian.

The Power of Openness and Inclusion in Countering Homophobia in Schools

by Tony Prince

When well-meaning teachers begin to address discrimination and harassment based on sexual orientation, their first impulse usually is to declare that they no longer will tolerate such words as "faggot" and "dyke" in their classrooms. I have spoken with teachers who proudly claim that they have declared their rooms "hate-free" zones. However, when I ask them what they are incorporating into their curriculum to educate students about people with different sexual orientations, almost uniformly they have been unable to cite even one instance of curricular inclusion.

These teachers are not creating "hate-free" zones; they are creating "speech-restriction" zones. While they may feel better that they no longer have to hear people call Johnny a "fag" and Julie a "dyke" every day, they probably are not creating meaningful change that will extend beyond the walls of their classrooms. Unless students have been genuinely educated with solid information about homosexuality and bisexuality and the real people who are and were what they are calling "fags" and "dykes," these students will have no reason not to want to name-call and almost certainly will engage in such behavior as soon as the teacher is not around to prevent it.

In fact, speech restrictions may create an even more hostile climate for gay and lesbian students by giving their bigoted peers the impression that they simply are not being allowed to express their opinions.

Forced squelching of bigoted speech continues to hide the real issues. Gay students do not need to be threatened and harassed, but they do need (and more and more frequently, demand) to be acknowledged. The alarming number of gay teen suicides surely indicates that the metaphorical closet of secrecy and shame makes schools scary and dangerous places for gay students. Yet in the vast majority of schools, homosexuality continues to remain hidden and therefore unaddressed. If teachers honestly want to be supportive of gay students and to increase the ease at which these young people can live and develop as happy and productive individuals, they will achieve that goal only by the infusion of accurate and representative information into the curriculum.

True inclusion affects all subjects.

Gay students need to understand and appreciate the contributions made by people like them as a way of validating their self-worth. The dissemination of this information also is essential in helping to lead their straight peers toward greater understanding, ultimately helping them to overcome their irrational desire to call gay students names or to beat them up.

When administrators look at the issue of gay and lesbian curriculum inclusion, their usual response is either to ignore the issue and hope that it will fade away or to relegate the issue to the health or sex education curriculum. The implication in the latter is that homosexuality is about sexual activity and its physical ramifications (usually characterized in terms of diseases and psychological problems) and not about history, literature, science, and every other field of academic study. Although accurate representation in the sex education and health curricula is essential, it is not the end-all of curricular inclusion. True inclusion affects all subjects.

Probably the most common method of inclusion currently used by teachers is that of mentioning the sexual orientation of famous gay, lesbian, and bisexual persons of note when those individuals are discussed during the natural course of teaching. However, there are many other ways in which information about homosexuality and homosexual persons can and should be shared with students. For example, in foreign language classes, students might select topics from a list of issues currently being debated in the United States and look at the various ways in which other countries deal with them. That list might include gay rights. Similarly, in social studies or history classes, the struggle for equal rights for gay men and lesbians should be addressed as a facet of civil rights.

English teachers have many options for inclusion. One of the more effective units that I have developed over the past few years with my sophomore classes is one that centers on the Essential Question (to use the Coalition of Essential Schools' lingo): Should males and females be treated equally? In this unit we begin by discussing the question is general terms. Every year virtually all of the students insist that their answer to this question is, always was, and always will be an unequivocal "yes." But then we look back to the 18th century and read, discuss, and write a brief essay about an excerpt from Mary Wollstonecraft's "A Vindication on the Rights of Women." We move on to the 19th century and Charlotte Perkins Gilman's short story, "If I Were a Man," in which a woman suddenly finds herself magically transformed into a man. The students are asked to imagine that they have been likewise transformed on the first day of school and to chronicle their impressions of that first day. Usually, issues involving sexual orientation begin to emerge during this assignment. In their stories, some students' sexual orientations change when their sex changes, while some maintain their interest in their current boy- or girlfriend. Sometimes students write amusingly about an erotic interest in their newly provided access to locker rooms.

Being thought to be a homosexual is the "worst thing" that many [students] can imagine.

This consideration leads to other questions: Should women be allowed to wear pants? Should men be allowed to wear dresses? Should women shave their legs and armpits and wear make-up? Should men? By this time, students are espousing views that contradict their original commitment to gender equality and are starting to question their own biases and presumptions.

Inevitably, it seems, many male students support inequities based on gender, saying that if those surface behavior boundaries are crossed, "people will think you're gay." Being thought to be a homosexual is the "worst thing" that many of them can imagine.

Little in this assignment directly addresses homophobia. Rather, it helps students think about sexual orientation issues, to dig beneath the surface and, in many cases, to discover the underpinnings of sexism, on which homophobia depends. Sexism and homophobia are closely related and mutually dependent.

31

I am convinced that educators have had only limited success in helping young people overcome sexist attitudes because we have not yet dealt with the homophobia that helps to maintains those attitudes. Until we address that link in our classrooms, we will continue to fail at our attempts to overcome sexism or homophobia.

One would think that being inclusive in one's curriculum in Kentucky would be simpler because of the Kentucky Education Reform Act (KERA). After all, that act was constructed by some of the most progressive educators in the country. It is intended to open up the schools for progress and innovation. It emphasizes critical thinking skills and personalization in the making of assignments. However, it has at least one major problem. It is built on the fragile premise that if teachers and parents are empowered to control the curriculum, the extracurricular activities, and even the use of building space, then dramatic, student-centered change is inevitable.

Unfortunately, when you throw an openly gay teacher into the mix, what do you get? In our school, the answer is a series of attempts to restrict students from having access to ideas and information that may contradict their, their parents', or even other faculty members' "beliefs." I even have been told by one parent that their family does not "believe in" homosexuality, as if this fact of human existence were a figment of the imagination that could be dismissed by their lack of belief.

Imagine the folly of "empowering" teachers, parents, and principals in Mississippi in the 1950s to make all decisions about their schools, including those involving African Americans, and you get some idea about the way in which gay issues are being addressed (or rather neglected and restricted) in Kentucky.

As of this writing, I am in the midst of a struggle with our site-based council over the availability and presentation of materials including gay people. Because the council, by law, may determine which instructional materials are to be taught in the school, they argue that they have complete autonomy to determine which materials might be "objectionable." We live in a climate of incredible fear, harassment, and intolerance; and I am very much afraid that the current trend toward site-based management that is now sweeping the country will make matters worse, particularly in the less-informed communities. Our council has appointed a "Materials Selection Subcommittee"

Jefferson County Public Schools has refused to include "sexual orientation" in the student code of conduct listing of areas in which harassment and name-calling are not permitted.

that has proposed a parent permission form for all materials that "may be controversial." Needless to say, this policy would prevent students of homophobic parents from getting any accurate information at all about gay men and lesbians.

However, as is typical of homophobic policies developed to disempower openly gay people, its scope and intent are not entirely clear. One of the problems with intentionally vague policies is that it is difficult for those they target to prove conclusively that the policies have a hostile intent. Ironically, this same vagueness makes them virtually unenforceable. After all, how can one draw the line to demarcate what "may be controversial" and thus necessitate special permission to teach and alternate assignments? Are alternate assignments to be required for skinheads when talking about black issues? For Christians when talking about Moslem or Jewish individuals?

Two years ago, as the commonwealth's only openly gay teacher, I was declared "significantly deficient" by my principal in my first year of teaching.* Last year, a senior student at another Louisville high school was told by his principal that he could not tell people at school that he is gay. The young man retaliated by wearing a dress to school to openly declare his homosexuality. He was not only suspended but also was arrested and jailed for "trespassing" when he refused to leave the school. Those who were taunting and threatening him received no disciplinary action. Since that time, although formally asked to do so by the Jefferson County Teachers Association and other individuals and organizations, Jefferson County Public Schools has refused to include "sexual orientation" in the student code of conduct listing of areas in which harassment and name-calling are not permitted.

In such a hostile climate, it is amazing that about a dozen other teachers and I have been able to establish a gay and lesbian teachers' caucus within our local National Education Association affiliate. Although none of the other teachers is open about his or her sexual orientation, the organization has sent a strong message of concern by its very existence. Immediately after the board of directors of the Jefferson County Teachers Association unanimously

---

*This experience is chronicled in detail in my chapter in Kevin Jennings' book, *One Teacher in Ten,* published by Alyson Press in 1994.

approved the formation and recognition of our caucus, a small group of teachers began to demand that the caucus be disbanded and its official status be withdrawn. Their attempts were unsuccessful, and the union officials maintained their support for us and continue to do so to this day.

Freedom of speech and the freedom to assemble peaceably are frightening to some people. I wish I could say that it is only our opponents who mistrust these constitutionally guaranteed freedoms, but I fear it is not. While our opponents were attempting to restrict our freedoms, several of our members, themselves closeted and refusing to speak publicly about the issue, were appallingly quick to criticize those who oppose us for exercising their right to speak out.

Clearly, all of us, both straight and gay, who are well-educated on sexual orientation issues need to inform and educate those who are not. Openness is never easy, especially when one is being open about an issue that has been long hidden. However, for gay educators, it will be only by speaking out clearly and persistently, both inside and outside the classroom, that we can raise and address the issues that affect gay and lesbian students and teachers. Opponents of gay and lesbian people must be allowed to voice their views, whether they are students, parents, teachers, administrators, or school board members. Ultimately, the powers of logic and reason will win out. Scores of social and scientific studies are on our side. The only way we can lose is if we squelch, hide, or run from the debate.

Coaching and Homosexuality

by Dan Woog

If you believe the research statistics, in my career I've coached two to three dozen gay soccer players. After all, I've been coaching soccer for nearly 20 years. With 15 to 18 new athletes a year, and the percentage of gay males estimated at somewhere between 5% and 10% of the population, that is one or two per team per year.

In all that time, not one boy has even hinted to me that he may be homosexual. In subsequent years, I have learned that several former players indeed are; some I've suspected, others I never would have imagined. I know there are many others I don't know about.

And in almost all that time, I never revealed my homosexuality to my players. They might have guessed — I'm unmarried, I live alone, I don't date women — and the older I got, the more the rumor mill probably perked. But I never brought it up, and no one else ever did either. On my soccer teams, "don't ask, don't tell" was alive and well.

Two years ago I finally came out of the closet — the locker room closet, as well as the many others I cowered in. My coming out vehicle was my weekly column in the *Westport* (Connecticut) *News*. (When I am not coaching soccer, I am a freelance writer.) A major impetus for my decision was the work I did on the athletic field. This is one coach's coming out story.

A long-term association with Staples High School's soccer program (one of the most successful in the nation; I played there before I coached there), 10 European tours as the organizer of successful soccer trips, my selection as National Youth Soccer Coach of the Year in 1990, and two decades as a national soccer writer, all combined to earn me the respect of my players, their parents, and my colleagues.

My coaching career taught me a great deal about adolescents: how they think, what they dream, who they are. Being around Staples High gave me good insight into high school education. And so during the 1993 March on Washington for Gay, Lesbian, and Bisexual Equal Rights and Liberation, I attended a reception hosted by the National Education Association. It was there that I met Sasha Alyson, whose Alyson Publications is the country's largest publisher of gay- and lesbian-themed books. We talked about potential book topics, and eventually we came up with the idea for *School's Out: The Impact of Gay and Lesbian Issues on America's Schools*, which was published in May 1995. (See Resources.)

As part of my research, I interviewed nearly 300 teachers, administrators, students, guidance counselors, nurses, support staff, and coaches. I spoke with Reggie Sellars, the openly gay assistant football coach at Noble and Greenough School in Dedham, Massachusetts, and to Katherine Henderson, assistant director of athletics and former volleyball and lacrosse coach at Phillips Andover Academy. They spoke movingly of the coming out process and how it affected not only them but also their athletes and, ultimately, their entire schools.

Reggie, for example, spoke of the easy acceptance of his revelation by his football team and how stunned he was when he realized that by fearing homophobia, he had stereotyped them just as ignorantly as he himself had been stereotyped as both a gay man and an African American. Kathy described her anxious hours between coming out to Andover (in an article for the school newspaper) and the subsequent team practice. She was overwhelmed to find that her athletes had decorated every volleyball and water bottle with supportive pink triangles, the symbol of gay and lesbian pride.

The more I spoke with these courageous men and women, the more I recognized that by not being out, I was doing all my soccer players — straight as well as gay — a disservice. Every afternoon at practice I preached honesty, yet every time I changed pronouns when discussing with whom I saw a movie or went to dinner, I lied. Every team member understood that I tolerated no racial, ethnic, or religious slurs, yet every one also knew I said nothing whenever anyone called someone else "gay" or used the word "fag." Every player looked up to me as a role model — for sportsmanship and fair play; for compassion as well as competition; for someone who stressed the importance of education and the arts along with athletics — yet in the area where I could be the most important role model of all, where I could prove that a man could be both macho and gay, I was frozen with fear.

But ever so slowly, I inched out of the closet door.

In February 1994 I gave a talk in our school library about my book. More than 300 students attended — more, I proudly tell people, than attended similar talks by noted authors Paul Kennedy and Richard Seltzer. (I harbor no illusions about why they came. Homosexuality is far more enticing to teenagers than international affairs or medicine.) I discussed the process of research, writing, and publishing as much as the content. But, of course, every question centered on gayness. I had promised myself that, if asked, I would say I was gay; however, no one dared to pop the question. Suburban boys and girls, I guess, are too polite.

After that meeting, several girls approached me with the idea of starting a gay/straight alliance. A straight teacher, Ann Friedman, agreed to work with me; and our principal, Gloria Rakovic, recognized that this fit right into her year-long theme of "diversity." Within weeks our group had about 20 regular members.

I grew more and more confident about coming out. I wrote a coming out column for the local paper; it was set to run on May 27. The day before, at our weekly Gay/Straight Alliance meeting, we chatted about what we'd accomplished in a few months of existence. Someone said, "I just feel bad no one's felt comfortable enough to come out at one of our meetings."

There was a brief pause, then I jumped in. "Pick up the paper tomorrow morning. Read my column," I said simply.

Instantly, they got it. One boy, sitting in the front row, stared at me with awe in his eyes. I knew I'd made the right decision.

The next morning I was nervous but excited. My column usually is well-read. This one, I knew, would be particularly so. I walked into the cafeteria — the student hangout — and felt a buzz in the air. Everyone had seen the column, yet no one had a clue what to say or how to act. I looked around. About 50 Stapleites either stared right at me or glanced quickly away.

. . . by not being out, I was doing all my soccer players — straight as well as gay — a disservice.

Suddenly Tim Caffrey — the popular and well-respected soccer captain — walked over and stuck out his hand. "Great column, Dan," he said. "I'm proud of you."

That broke the ice. For the rest of the day, students approached me. Some complimented me on my column; others patted my arm as they walked by. A few just smiled — friendly, not mocking smiles. I made contact with people I'd never spoken to before. I learned about gay and lesbian relatives, so many that I felt like saying, "Okay, if you want to talk about an aunt or uncle, line up here; a cousin, over there; if it's a parent or sibling, I'll talk to you right now."

If the T-shirt that made its way to the top of my drawer and then into my gym bag happened to be one from the San Francisco Gay Pride parade of 1991, I wore it.

The good feeling continued for days, with the soccer players among the most enthusiastic. Congratulations poured in. Current players spoke to me in person, while former players called, wrote letters, and, this being the 1990s, sent E-mail messages. "It's cool" was the gist of what most conveyed. You're a good coach, we like you, and now we know a little bit more about you.

Only two parents called, and both were complimentary. One man said my column had allowed him to have "the kind of honest discussion with [his son] that every father wishes he could have." Another said, in a similar vein, that that night they had "the best dinner table conversation ever." Both ended their calls the same way: "Thanks for coaching my son."

I expected soccer people to be, if not accepting, at least not intolerant. After all, the game attracts a certain type of creative, intelligent, worldly person. I was less sure about the reaction of athletes and coaches in other sports. Yet they also went out of their way to let me know that, even if they did not delight in the news or want it for themselves or family members, it did not change our relationship one bit. Football, basketball, baseball, and lacrosse players complimented me on my "guts" (now there's an athletic metaphor!); coaches said that it gave them a bit more insight into the person I am. The closest I got to a negative response came from a football coach, who happened to be reading my piece the same time I walked past his office. "Hey," he said immediately. "If that's what you are, and that's what you want, it's fine with me." I could not have asked for more from him.

The fall season began. I did not stand on a soapbox, preaching about homosexuality and homophobia, demanding tolerance and respect when I should have been teaching passing and shooting, but neither did I shy away from the subject. If someone asked why there was no practice on a certain Friday, I told them: I was at the National Lesbian and Gay Journalists Association convention. If the T-shirt that made its way to the top of my drawer and then into my gym bag happened to be one from the San Francisco Gay Pride parade of 1991, I wore it. And if a player wandered, inadvertently or not, onto the rocky terrain of gay issues, I met him there.

One day a boy tried to explain why a certain teammate was disliked. "It's always been that way," he said. "Even when we were in elementary school, we had a TIAF Club."

"What's that?" I asked innocently.

Suddenly the player looked stricken. He opened his mouth but was literally unable to speak.

"Come on," I prodded. "It can't be that bad. What is it?"

Finally, without looking me in the eye, he mumbled, "Tom Is A Fag."

"Well," I said, "I appreciate you telling me. Kind of makes you think about the power of words, doesn't it?" At last, grateful to be let off the hook, he looked at me and nodded.

Another time, the varsity was shaking hands after a tough win over a big rival. "Faggot," one opponent said as he went through the line. The boy whose hand he was shaking had outplayed him, and in his frustration that was all he could say.

I reacted immediately. "No, I don't think he is," I said to the opponent. "I am; he's not." The stunned boy just stared. He had no idea how to respond. The players on our team roared and high-fived me. We'd won more than the game.

In 1995, in what is believed to be the first event of its kind anywhere, I presented a workshop on "Homosexuality, Homophobia, and Soccer" at the National Soccer Coaches Association of America (NSCAA) 48th annual convention in Washington, D.C. Although the convention itself drew a record 3,500 college and high school coaches, the homophobia workshop attracted only 75. That number did not disappoint me. I'm sure many coaches did not attend because they were worried about being seen, and a workshop at the same time featuring the national team coach drew many others. But the ones who came proved what I've always believed. This is an important topic that must be talked about. Getting 75 people to discuss homophobia in sports was a great step forward.

The Moonie-owned *Washington Times* had predicted my presentation would be the most controversial of the entire convention and quoted one person as wondering why the topic needed addressing at all. "It's a bit like a talk on the Bosnian conflict at a shoe salesman's conference," the anonymous coach said. I had told the reporter I disagreed with that quote, saying, "If we coaches are truly the people we say we are — teachers and educators concerned about the physical and emotional growth of every person we coach, straight and gay — then this is a topic we cannot ignore." But he chose not to print that.

In fact, the entire newspaper piece was decidedly negative; but I used that to my advantage in the introduction. "I could say, 'What do you expect from a paper owned by the Moonies?' — but I won't," I began. "That would stereotype every Moonie based on what I've heard, not what I know. There might even be Moonies in the audience — I don't know who you are or what you look like. That might embarrass you, if you don't want your Moonie-ality made public. After all, most people in America don't like Moonies; they don't want their kids coached by them, and they certainly don't want them to grow up to *be* Moonies." The audience understood the parallel to stereotyping gay men and lesbians.

I had hoped to put together a workshop involving several openly gay coaches and athletes, nicely balanced between gender, age, and geographic area. What I found, while trying to arrange such an event, was that those people who were willing to talk were unable to come to Washington, while those who were able to be there were unwilling to speak publicly. So I gathered four life stories and presented them myself. All were true, and the athletes and coaches were eager that their tales be told, even though they had various reactions to using their names and schools.

Chris, a former player at a major Southern university, is a distant relative of Jesse Helms. ("I'd be even more distant if he knew I was gay," he joked.) As a college freshman he did not come out because he feared being kicked off the team. "I didn't want to jeopardize our chances of winning over something as inconsequential to me — but big to other people — as my sexuality," he said.

But as a sophomore he did come out, to the surprise of everyone. Some team members told him they'd continue to play soccer together, but that socializing off the field was out. Others said it was no problem. One night Chris took a few of them to a gay bar, and they all had a great time. The on-field support even took the form of a few strategic fouls against opponents who taunted Chris.

Chris felt his decision to come out to his teammates was a good one. "It was very self-satisfying to live my life fully," he said, "and maybe I opened the eyes of some homophobic people." In the three months after he came out, five people came out to him. "They saw I could be macho and gay," he analyzed.

Chris's advice to straight players about dealing with a gay teammate, or one who is rumored to be gay, is, "Be self-assured. I may be attracted to a straight person, but I know not to do anything stupid. I can't be converted to heterosexuality, and you can't be converted to homosexuality."

Morgan Robinson's teenage years in a Boston suburb were not easy. Because he was "different," he was teased, even on the soccer field. But, he said, "I went through crap for 10 years because I loved the game."

He loved it enough to be picked for the Massachusetts state team, and when he transferred to private Concord Academy, he found his niche. He became a four-year varsity player and was twice elected captain.

He came out as bisexual to the entire school during "chapel," a 15-minute block of time in which any senior can speak. "I blew the school away," he recalled. "I was captain of the soccer team, with a big reputation for dating girls."

But no one was fazed by his announcement. "Terrific chapel," his coach said. "Now let's get back to work." Part of that reaction was because he was known as an easy-going person; part was the respect he'd earned as a player and leader. "Good players don't get picked on," he noted.

Morgan currently is involved in Boston's City Year volunteer program as an HIV/AIDS peer educator. He plans to play soccer next year in college.

Kelly Wheeler never came out in high school or college because, she said, "I didn't have the depth of understanding to know there was a life for lesbians to live. I had no idea how a lesbian would fit in with her community, her family. I was just so fearful of the repercussions in society and on my team." So she dated men.

Her Ithaca College team was close-knit and good. They won an NCAA Division III national championship her junior year. Still, Kelly did not come out. Today — with the knowledge that several other teammates also are lesbians — she regrets it.

"Why can't you just let it be?"

"My teammates would've supported me, and I would have been able to progress a little farther," she said. "I would have had more honest, long-lasting friendships with my teammates. And that's the value of athletics: going through hard times together, so the bonds will endure long after college."

But, she noted, everyone has her own timing and process for accepting herself. Hers brought her to the end of college; she did not deal with her sexuality until she moved to Colorado and had time and space to think. She's now a physical therapist there and says she is happier than she's ever been.

As far as lesbians in soccer generally, Kelly said, "There will be lesbians on any team, just like in any classroom. And we don't all look butch, either. In fact, our soccer team was so well-rounded, good looking, and 'feminine,' no one could believe we won a national championship!"

Mark McGrath came out at the private Dwight-Englewood School in New Jersey soon after the team he helped coach won the county championship. "I was teaching [history and law] and coaching well, and kids were responding to that," he said. "I had success and the support of my peers." Head coach Chris Schmid — "a stout, macho German," Mark called him — was particularly accepting.

His players had no inkling he was gay. After his announcement, no one changed for the worse. In fact, Mark found that some sought him out more — to discuss personal issues. A few players even joined a gay and straight student alliance group that he helped to form.

He knows that not all schools are like Dwight-Englewood, and he knows from comments he hears that homophobia does exist in soccer. However, he said, "I give soccer people a lot of credit for being more open than other sports. Soccer lends itself to acceptance. It's a team game in which players have to rely on each other. It's a game in which players teach themselves — and people who think on their own tend to be able to analyze situations objectively. It's an international game, and generally homophobia is less rampant overseas than it is here. It's a game in which people are free to be who they are."

His final comment was: "When I went to the coaches' convention, no matter what city it was in, I never failed to see other coaches at the local gay bar."

One of those coaches then addressed the Washington workshop. He was active in the Gay Games and is an officer in the International Lesbian and

As an openly gay soccer coach, I am happier, healthier, even more successful, both on the field and off, than I ever have been.

Gay Football (Soccer) Organization. He spoke honestly — with a bit of trepidation — of the reasons he was not out on his campus. He was not ready, he said, to confront his homophobic athletic director, nor did he know how his players would react. He regretted, however, not being able to help — as an advisor or simply as a role model — the players he suspects are gay.

There were many questions after our presentation. One man said, "I coach at the high school level. Doesn't a girl going on to college have the right not to play for a lesbian coach and not to play with lesbian teammates?"

"Let's turn that question around," I said. "Would you get up in a meeting like this and say, 'Doesn't a girl have the right not to play for a black coach, or with Hispanic teammates?'

"Furthermore, what happens if she chooses a college because she thinks the coach is not a lesbian and that there are no lesbian players? When she graduates and gets a job, chances are she'll have lesbian co-workers — maybe even a lesbian boss. How is she going to be able to get along with them if she hasn't learned those lessons earlier?

"The issue is not whether she has to play with lesbian teammates or for a lesbian coach, but rather why that's a problem for her," I concluded.

The next questions came from an athletic director. "I understand all that you're saying," he began, "but why do you have to talk about it? Why can't you just let it be?"

My answer was that the issue is there whether it's talked about or not, so it is better to bring it into the open than to bury it. "If a player on your team shuts himself off from his teammates because he's scared, they'll find out his secret; you're not going to have the best team possible," I said. "And if you've got something that is tearing the team apart, you're not going to be a very effective coach."

Another man wondered about pedophilia. "I'm glad you brought that up," I replied. "I'm worried, too. I'm worried about the 5% of pedophilia acts that are committed by gay men, and the 95% that are committed by straight men — most of whom are married. I think we all have to be concerned about every person who is coaching every boy and girl."

It was a good ending to a remarkable day. Several dozen coaches had their eyes opened, their horizons broadened. There was plenty of information presented and lots of honest give-and-take. My only surprise was that no one approached me afterward and came out — either as gay or as a Moonie.

Which brings us to the present. The Staples High School Gay/Straight Alliance continues to meet weekly. We are attracting more and more students from all corners of the high school. The longer we exist, the deeper we are integrated into the fabric of the school — and the less often we find our posters defaced. Coming out has freed me as a writer to become both bolder and more honest. That is not a guess; several students have told me, "Dan, your columns are getting really good!"

As an openly gay soccer coach, I am happier, healthier, even more successful, both on the field and off, than I ever have been. I have the respect of my athletes and colleagues and, more important, I respect myself. At long last the themes that I have for so long tried to convey in my twin careers of writing and coaching — honesty, integrity, being true to oneself — are part of my own life, too.

Part Two
Curricular Issues

The Case for a Gay and Lesbian Curriculum*

by Arthur Lipkin

Introduction: The Political Context

For a short time recently the debate about New York's "Children of the Rainbow Curriculum" was a rallying point for public discourse about the nature of sexuality and families. The battle over the inclusion of gay-positive instruction in a broad multicultural curriculum evinced a homophobic barrage from a multiethnic chorus, informed with religious zealotry and other biases of the Right. Some reporters observed a diversion of troops from family-planning clinics to school yards.

For gay progressives the Rainbow controversy was the first national arena in which to take on social conservatives on the issue of education. For those who see schools as a crucial site for anti-oppression education and for social change, the New York engagement held the promise of being a Stonewall for the Nineties. They understand that getting at the roots of homophobia requires more than the public relations campaigns prescribed by some critics within the gay community (Kirk and Madsen 1989; Stafford 1988); it re-

*This article first appeared in *The High School Journal* 77, nos. 1 and 2 (October-November 1993/December-January 1994), pp. 95-107. Reprinted with permission of the author and the publisher.

quires early intervention, conscientious curriculum change, programmatic staff development, and student support. Though some may have strategic differences with their cohorts in New York, they welcomed the clash over the Rainbow as a first significant and possibly galvanizing engagement in their campaign to remake schools into gay-supportive environments.

Unfortunately for these progressives, an historical accident made military service the temporary focal point of the struggle for gay rights. The campaign to lift the military ban diverted national attention from the schools. "Heather's Two Mommies" lost their news billing to "Gays in Uniform." But with the military issue at least temporarily settled, attention can turn again to the matter of Rainbow curricula. And, in re-focusing on schools, we ought to be reminded that the adult antagonists in all national debates about civil rights and diversity have spent a considerable part of their formative years in schools where their understandings of human differences might have been enhanced.

Why Teach These Things?

We can justify teaching about homosexuality on pragmatic as well as scholarly grounds. Since our schools have both social and intellectual objectives, it should be satisfying to ground this reform firmly in both arenas.

One practical reason that the subject of homosexuality is appropriate, especially for high school students, is that they find the topic engaging. Indeed, the entire realm of sexuality can be an obsession for adolescents. One may argue that the mass media contribute to the exaggeration of this aspect of human experience for young people. But even without the commodification of sex — the suasions of MTV, teen magazines, film, and advertising — the protracted coming-of-age process that has developed in our culture would probably find sexual musings and anxieties at its core. Today's students are not only thinking and talking; they are "doing" sexuality at a high rate and at a very young age (Haignere 1987; Zelnik and Shah 1983). If schools are going to have any impact on the attitudes and behaviors of their sexually concerned and often active students, they must acknowledge in their curricula the importance of sexuality in our lives and in the lives of those who have

Americans are embarrassed to admit their interest in sexual representations because they fear their curiosity makes them immoral.

gone before us. This academic exercise will not only illuminate the details of sexuality; it will also put it in perspective.

Americans are embarrassed to admit their interest in sexual representations because they fear their curiosity makes them immoral. For example, they would rather see explicit sex on screen than see violence, but they assume their neighbors would prefer the opposite. Researchers who study this contradiction between natural interest and shame believe that people's notions of public morality have been skewed by the outspokenness of religious conservatives (Donnerstein et al. 1993). The widespread perception that sexual interest is uncommon and sinful may be corrected by including realistic, developmentally appropriate, sex education curricula in schools.

Sexual ignorance in our culture can be a strong rationale for teaching sex education in general, but what about homosexuality in particular? On the practical level, what is it about homosexuality that provokes the interest of students? Adolescents appear to be as much obsessed with conformity as they are with sex. At the same time a youth discovers his individual sexuality, he is also intent on conforming to peer group norms. Our culture makes the very personal exploration of sexuality into a process of self-definition in a comparative context. Is it any wonder then, that not merely sexuality, but sexuality *difference* is a compelling concern for our young people?

What are the practical results of ignorance about sexuality differences? We must answer that question vis a vis each of two constituencies: those youth who are lesbian, gay, bisexual, or confused about their sexual interests and developing identities and those who are heterosexually identified.

Help for Gay Youth

The litany of stresses and self-inflicted injuries suffered by gay and struggling youth should be familiar: alienation, depression, substance abuse, and suicide (Hetrick and Martin 1987, 1988; Gonsiorek 1988; Hunter and Schaecher 1987; U.S. Dept. of Health and Human Services 1989; Remafedi, 1987, 1990).

It is hard to believe that any gay kid growing up listening to Phil Donahue, Oprah, or any other of the daily American cavalcade of afternoon TV could still feel isolated or think that he or she is the only one. The openness and variety of television discourses on sexuality must have some positive impact, but there is also a worrisome effect. The often sensationalistic nature of television talk programming indicates the currency of ratings over accuracy. The images of gay people on these shows could confuse or frighten the ordinary gay kid who might relate to neither the "motorcycle dyke" nor the "gay weight-lifter/model."

Second, an almost universal principle of TV talk on homosexuality, the inclusion of opposing views, is problematic. Having a guest with a different opinion usually means inviting a rabid homophobe. What message does the gay or confused youth take from a show that promotes the expression of undisguised bigotry?

Even a balanced and civil television presentation may evoke discouraging consequences. Though Phil and Oprah themselves often demonstrate an accepting attitude, how many voices of support in the life of the young gay viewer are raised as a result of the TV program? Parents or others may express negative views of homosexuality in response to the presentation. Classmates may do the same the next day in school. How many teachers are prepared or willing to conduct an impromptu class discussion? And how many of those teachers who pick up the buzz among students and react to it will express a tolerant view? Young gays' and lesbians' self-esteem is vitally linked to these sources of approval (Savin-Williams 1990; Weinberg 1983).

News and public affairs programming can also send alienating and dangerous messages to gay kids. The recent hearing on gays in the military, for instance, provided a stream of testimony that portrayed homosexuality, if not gay people, in a negative light. There was almost no testimony to counter the image of gays as predatory, infected, and incapable of promoting group solidarity or providing leadership. Coverage of the HIV epidemic is also skewed. The demography of AIDS in this country insures that most AIDS programming focuses on gay men.

There are exceptions to these characterizations of homosexuality on television. There is the occasional objective discussion, a flattering or good-humored portrayal, and, rarely, an average gay citizen actually speaking about his or her own life. But, for the most part, mass media conflate homosexuality with controversy and suffering. Exposed to these images, gay youth, especially those in remote areas, must have a dismal view of their prospects. Indeed one wonders if these young people experience their sexuality much differently from the way most gay people did fifty years ago. Without exposure to a vibrant urban gay community and without the support of family, friends, or school, gay youth can be deeply bruised by these media messages.

Gay/lesbian/bisexual and struggling students can be helped by bringing the discussion of gay issues into the school. All of the researchers who have studied homosexual identity formation have described a developmental stage in which these people consider what they know about gayness to see if the label is congruent with what they know about themselves (Herdt 1989; Coleman 1988; Troiden 1988; Cass 1984). If they are aware only of a limited number of features of gay life, they may have difficulty in this process of identification. Since many conceptions of homosexuality in our society are inaccurate and stigmatizing, gay youth may rightfully fear the burden they are taking upon themselves. These are the conflicts and feelings of alienation from their developing identities that cause gay teens to harm themselves (Herdt and Boxer 1993).

On the other hand, if gay youth are exposed to the diversity of gay identities, to the richness of the culture, and to the long history of same-gender attraction, their development will be enhanced. That is not to say that the homosexual experience ought to be so glamorized that unrealistic expectations will be fostered. However, students should learn that there is more to celebrate in being gay than there may be to fear. We have plenty of evidence in gay history and literature, as well as in current events, that the gay experience, like that of other minorities, is fraught with risk. But for students who are gay, lesbian, or bisexual, developing a balanced and accurate view of what it can mean to be gay could literally save their lives.

Needless to say, gay youth will also benefit from any increase in tolerance that results from greater understanding. Violence against gay people has a long history and appears to be increasing since the advent of AIDS and growing public expressions of homophobia related to political questions. The perpetrators of violence against gays and lesbians are most often young men (Levin and McDevitt 1993; Herek and Berill 1992).

It should come as no surprise then that high schools are a frequent site for homophobic rage and violence.

. . . if gay youth are exposed to the diversity of gay identities, to the richness of the culture, and to the long history of same-gender attraction, their development will be enhanced.

51

Help for Heterosexual Youth

School programs about homosexuality help gay youth with their adjustment. In fact, most such programs are conceived for that purpose. The recent report of the Governor's Commission on Gay and Lesbian Youth in Massachusetts is titled *Making Schools Safe for Gay and Lesbian Youth* (1993). Perhaps the first such state-sponsored effort in the country, this laudable report calls on schools to be sensitive to the needs of gay youth, to prevent the harm these students do to themselves, and to curb the violence that is often directed at them.

Implicit in the Massachusetts report and others like it (Seattle Commission 1988; McManus, et al. 1991; Schoenhals 1992) is the unspoken notion that gay youth will be the only beneficiaries of the recommendations. It is crucial to this effort, however, to acknowledge the benefits to heterosexual people of a better understanding of homosexuality.

First, it can be argued that any learning that eliminates prejudice not only helps its target but also frees the bigot himself from victimization. Hate is a debilitating burden to carry around; letting go of prejudice, on the other hand, allows a stunted mind to grow to a more inclusive understanding of the human experience. This was a consequence ignored by the *Brown* v. *Board of Education* decision. Perhaps because it was ruling on the grievances of blacks in a separate and unequal system, the court limited itself to the observation that such separation harmed the black students' interests. It did not point out that lack of contact with black people resulted in a poor education for whites. Segregation hindered the white child's understanding of the breadth of human experience by limiting his contact with his black neighbor. Integration can prevent that by stimulating new dialogues about race. And that discourse can lead to unforeseen recasting of the meanings of race itself.

Getting over homophobia, the misunderstanding, fear, or hatred of homosexuality, can have direct benefits as well, analogous to those of a racially integrated education. Antihomophobia education can help heterosexual people to better understand their own sexualities. The requirements of heterosexual identity in our culture are narrow and rigid. Much anxiety is created over the need to live up to these requirements; and too many young people, especially young women, are hurt in the process. Learning about the range of expression of different sexualities can take some of the pressure off these students.

Ironically, understanding homosexuality, which is one extreme of sexuality in the Kinsey sense, may give people at the other extreme more latitude. The heterosexual student may recognize that he shares none of the homosexual experience and is not gay, or he may accept the homoerotic feelings he has experienced as nonthreatening to his heterosexuality, or he may come to believe that sexuality labels are arbitrary markers on a continuum. One heterosexually identified student recently expressed his new view after studying a unit on the history of gays and lesbians in the United States:

> The more we talk about homosexuality in class, the more comfortable I am with the idea, with gay people, with my own sexuality, and with my own male identity. Is/Was this curriculum and these discussions important? About as important as the desegregation of schools in the 50s and the abolition of slavery in the 1800s. We are in the *middle* of a *huge* societal movement, a tremendous change, one more step to a better society. (white male public high school senior, 1992)

Presenting homosexuality without embarrassment or condemnation signals a teacher's acceptance of sexuality in general. That attitude may facilitate important communication with heterosexual students. Openly gay and lesbian teachers have told how heterosexual students have come to them to discuss sexuality and relationship issues that they would not discuss with others. These students explained that they chose the gay teachers to talk to because they perceived them to be more understanding of different people's sexual experiences than they thought others would be (Ferreira et al. 1993).

What Can Schools Do?

Schools can have an impact on how students construe differences among them. In the areas of racial, ethnic, and gender difference the mere presence of visible minority group members in a school can lead to experiences and conversations that promote greater understanding. With the addition of a multicultural curriculum, learning about these kinds of differences is greatly enhanced.

But sexuality differences are more problematic. First, there are many communities where religious, moral, or political objections prevent teaching about homosexuality. And even where such barriers are absent, the likelihood of gay/lesbian/bisexual students or teachers being open about their sexuality is small. Pressure to remain closeted persists; therefore opportunities to interact with openly gay people in school activities are rare, as is learning about the gay experience informally from people who are part of the school community. Most schools who commit to inclusion of gays under the rubric of multiculturalism have to depend on a deliberate curriculum and guest speakers.

Antihomophobia education can help heterosexual people to better understand their own sexualities.

As has been illustrated in New York, gay curriculum seems even more controversial than gay civil rights. Because children are directly involved, stereotype-based hysteria rises quickly. Public figures want to avoid the accusation of "teaching kids how to be a homosexual" that inevitably flies whenever curriculum is suggested. In fact, during the New York battle, the curriculum recommendations of the Governor's Commission on Gay and Lesbian Youth in Massachusetts were quietly dropped from its report, as it made its way from the governor to the state's commissioner of education. On 20 May 1993 the front-page headline in the *Boston Herald* read, "There'll be no gay school lessons"; and the governor was quoted as saying, "I don't personally favor teaching a gay and lesbian curriculum in the schools."

Some level of controversy may be avoided by interpreting the notion of curriculum broadly. At a minimum the forbidding of homophobic name-calling (a part of the Massachusetts plan) is the beginning of curriculum. It implies the teaching of the value of tolerance in a particular context. Some in Massachusetts appear to believe that a teacher or administrator can ask a student not to call another "faggot" without having to explain who is being harmed by such language and why it is wrong to defame those people. Enforcement of a name-calling policy without explanation is shortsighted. The rule is important in setting a tone for the school and can create some value dissonance within the offender. But if the only rationale for the rule is the seemingly arbitrary authority of the school, then the behavior will likely be stopped only in the school. It may be resumed on the street.

If the name-calling rule is contextualized within a fairness discussion in which gay/lesbian people are given their humanity and misperceptions are challenged, tolerance may be internalized and practiced beyond the schoolhouse walls.

The next level of curriculum is the general sensitivity unit in which students are taught explicitly that they should be nice to gay people. Usually included with other kinds of difference, the category of homosexual may also be considered separately.

Though it may seem safer to include gays and lesbians in a larger litany of minority groups when teaching respect for differences, that approach can have its limitations. Despite the importance of mentioning gays in lessons on tolerance, teachers must also be prepared to discuss gay issues separately. Explicit classroom reference to gays is rare enough that students will naturally be inquisitive about their inclusion. Some students, particularly members of other minority groups, may not understand or may even resent the apparent equating of the minority statuses. Thoughtful amplification is required then, both to avoid glib superficiality and to clarify similarities and differences among oppressions.

Teachers should also be ready for questions to arise about their own sexuality. This phenomenon of thinking a teacher might be gay because he or she consistently includes gay people in the American patchwork is common. Raising the topic of racial oppression does not ordinarily lead to questions about a teacher's racial identity, since racial identity is usually apparent. Mention of religious or ethnic topics could generate assumptions about the teacher, but it is doubtful that they would have the same impact unless the community is sensitive to certain of those categories. Sexuality usually does provoke speculation, particularly if the teacher is not known to be married. Because of the pervasiveness of homophobia in our country and the accurate perception that gay people are the most active in the struggle against it, one who repeatedly defends gays is assumed to be homosexual.

Teachers should be prepared to do three things as a consequence of raising homosexual issues in the classroom. The first is to answer some basic questions about gayness, concerning: its prevalence, its possible causes, and its practices and cultural features. Second, the teacher must be able to point out features common to different forms of oppression, as well as the differences among minority groups' experiences. Third, teachers should be ready to respond comfortably to questions about their own sexualities . Stereotypes may be challenged effectively if the heterosexual teacher withholds information about his orientation until he has asked his students how they might feel differently about him if he were gay.

When gay/lesbian teachers raise issues of homosexuality with their students, there can be powerful repercussions. If these teachers are unwilling or forbidden to be open with students, their hiding can send a message of shame that is not conducive to healthy adolescent development. On the other hand, the gay teacher must have support in the school to undertake an admittedly problematical disclosure. There is no universal answer to this dilemma. In the end, no teacher, gay or heterosexual, should share intimate details of his erotic life with students; however, openness about sexual orientation can be part of a valuable lesson.

Beyond Sensitivity

No one should underestimate the value of teachers' including gay people when they talk with students about cultural diversity. For young people just to hear the words "homosexuality" or "gay/lesbian/bisexual" in an accepting context sends a powerful message and creates the potential for a tolerant environment. Further, when teachers are willing and able to discuss some basic facts of homosexuality and gay life, that potential is greatly increased.

But there are still limits to what these minimal curriculum strategies can accomplish. Urging students to be tolerant of gays along with other minorities, spending a few class minutes countering a handful of misconceptions, or even having a special "sensitivity session" about homophobia separates the gay experience from the central curricular goals of the school. The gesture could take on the characterization of a "politically correct" thing to do. We cannot deny the political nature of such inclusion nor, I would hope, its rectitude. But we should avoid giving it the aura of a trendy sideshow, conducted apart from the serious business of inquiry in our daily classes. A school rule about name-calling, the direct objection to homophobic harassment, mention of gays as a legitimate minority group, a multicultural awareness day featuring a segment on gays and lesbians — all these worthy steps should not relieve the school of its obligation to do more.

What is required is sustained and serious academic discourse within the disciplines of the school. Students need to understand the nature of sexual identity, the long history of same-gender attraction, and how it has been expressed in different times and cultures. They should know about past and current etiological research. They need to analyze how the homosexuality of a historical figure or an author might have influenced his or her life or work.

They need to know something about the history of the gay/lesbian community in the United States and current issues in gay life. They must appreciate the diversity of gays and lesbians in this country and around the world.

For many years, schools, in their zeal to transmit our common culture, have scanted the experiences and contributions of racial minorities. Homosexuality has been completely ignored. References, even to the gay liberation movement in the 1960s and 1970s, are almost nonexistent in high school U.S. history texts (Licata 1980-81). Ironically, unlike other minorities, many white gay people are featured in history and gay authors are read, but their sexuality and its implications are not mentioned. If our mission is to cultivate our students' interest in the truth and to give them the skills to begin the search for it, this kind of intentional ignorance runs counter to our goal. It may be that, some years ago, we could honestly say that scholarship was spotty on the subject of homosexuality and good sources of material were not available. Today the thriving pursuit of gay studies in the universities provides volumes of respected research and exciting theory. Our work is to make some of this new learning available to secondary school students.

Health and Sex Education

One caveat must be given before exploring the possibilities of gay content in the various subject areas. That is the danger of medicalization. Mention of homosexuality, if there is any, is most often done in the context of health and HIV curricula. Although it is perfectly appropriate to discuss some aspects of homosexuality in these venues, there is a strong possibility that students' views will be distorted in the process. We run the risk of having them think that homosexuality is inevitably linked with deviance and illness. Even if the teacher is gay-friendly and the curriculum is accurate, placing the matter under the subject heading of "health" or "disease prevention" carries its own message.

The consequences of medicalizing homosexuality can be negative for all students, but we ought to be particularly concerned about what gay/lesbian youth might experience. Any school that focuses exclusively on the physiological dimensions of homosexuality compounds the societal misconception

Presenting the ways that gay men and lesbians construct alternative families will generate opportunities for learning about aspects of gay life.

that gayness is just about sex acts. It objectifies the gay youth into a biological subject, reducing his experience in the world to his sex life. To be sure, sex education in general can result in the same distortion, regardless of the sexuality under consideration. However, curricular representations of heterosexual life outside the health class, in history and literature, for example, offset this effect by countering the impression with other facets of male-female relationships that are not only physical. For the gay student, this curricular balancing is, for the most part, absent.

In the case of AIDS education, gay students can benefit from knowledge that leads to less risk taking. Still, a school that examines homosexuality only in the shadow of a tragic illness offers little affirmation to its gay students. It is a struggle to make AIDS education positive for gay adults, many of whom have access to support within the gay community. It is even more difficult to reach gay youth, who lack community ties, with an AIDS message that affirms their sexuality.

In the area of family life curricula, there is a greater possibility than in health for a broader view of gay experience. Presenting the ways that gay men and lesbians construct alternative families will generate opportunities for learning about aspects of gay life such as spousal relationships, child-rearing, extended biological and intentional family, work-sharing, and financial planning.

Like learning about the range of sexuality itself, learning about how gay people make a family can have a positive, if not liberating, effect on heterosexual students, for whom normative definitions of family might prevent full human development. Young heterosexual women especially could benefit from understanding that there are other ways to thrive beyond conventional marriage. Of course, healthy models of unconventional family life may be provided by heterosexuals, too. Still, strong challenges to conservative notions of gender role may often be found in same-gender partnerships.

Family life education offers a natural place for the integration of gay content into standard courses, which is crucial for the success of gay studies in high schools. Courses in gay studies alone are not advisable. On a practical level, who would enroll in an independent gay-themed course? Two types of student who might most benefit from information in such classes would probably stay away. Gay or lesbian students who are not open about their sexuality would likely not enroll for fear of the stigma; and homophobic heterosexual students would probably not cross the threshold.

Furthermore, if we want to teach that gay people are a part of the community and the gay experience is a part of our cultural heritage, gay studies must not be segregated. We must underscore the value to all students of learning about these things. It is too easy for schools to ghettoize minority studies and the people who enroll in them. School authorities can cover their bases in what they may see as a multicultural game; but in so doing, they suppress the truth of our national life, which has always been multicultural.

Social Studies

The social studies present fertile ground for the integration of a gay curriculum, particularly in the disciplines of history, political science, sociology, anthropology, and psychology. Of primary interest in these areas are: cross-cultural and transhistorical understandings and representations of same-gender sexuality; the importance of certain gay/lesbian people in various eras; the evolution of the modern gay identity; current gay issues, including legal rights, medicine, activism, and politics.

An eight- to ten-day curriculum, "The Stonewall Riots and the History of Gays and Lesbians in the U.S.," will serve as an example of a social studies unit. Used effectively in both U.S. history and sociology classes in the Cambridge, Massachusetts, public high school, the unit begins with colorful accounts, taken from contemporary newspapers, of the 1969 riots at the Stonewall Inn, a gay bar in Greenwich Village. Beginning a study of gay history with this event pulls students into a vivid conflict. They are then asked to consider such questions as: Who were these people? Why were they there? Had there always been gay people in New York? What is the significance of this event historically — was it a turning point in our national awareness? How does it compare with other historical events of a similar nature? The unit then recapitulates the history of same-gender expression from the Colonial Period through the present, with special attention to urbanization, the impact of the World Wars, and the ascendancy of science. Economically and racially diverse groups of students have studied this unit from 1991 to 1993. The following are selected observations from their final exams (excerpted verbatim):

I came in thinking I knew at least something about the gay movement, because I know many people who are gay. Yet I knew barely anything about the Stonewall incident. (White female)

It is good that people organize a group to help teach kids to understand the values and feelings of gays and lesbians, so they might understand them and know that they too are humans. (Hispanic male)

I have always thought what people do is their business, but it has taught me that society and its rules for "norms" can do a job on a group of people. (White female)

It is very similar to the Black Civil Rights Movement. That helps me understand the movement more. The lesson also helped me to be open-minded to homosexuals. (African-American female)

I was aware that the gay rights movement is still going on. I have always at least within the last couple of years had a concern for human rights. I did know that homosexuals have been around for hundreds of years. In this class I learned the history of homosexual identity. (White male)

The routine un-sensationalized inclusion of homosexual possibilities in the high school curriculum would have a profoundly positive effect.

A three- to five-day unit, "The History and Nature of Homosexuality and Its 'Causes'," has been used for three years in biology classes in Cambridge. It is appropriate to psychology classes as well. This unit examines the changing understandings of same-gender desire from ancient Greece to contemporary America. More detailed observations than those in the Stonewall unit are made concerning the changes brought about by developments in science and medicine. Recent psychological and biological theories of etiology are explained. One theme of this unit is the influence of culture and politics on scientific inquiry.

Literature

The question of what is meant by "gay literature" or the "gay aesthetic" has not been answered yet. What may be said here is that the influence of a gay writer's sexuality on his or her work is worth examining in high school English, foreign language, or world literature classes. The pantheon of writers who invite this analysis include both well-known gay writers such as Auden, Baldwin, Forster, Williams, Woolf, Cather, Whitman, Wilde, Gide, and Verlaine, whose works are already part of the secondary school canon, and those, perhaps lesser known, who could be taught successfully in high schools (Radcliffe Hall, Isherwood, Vivien, Leavitt, Mishima, Renault, etc.).

There are other writers whose sexualities are subject to debate. Some of them figure prominently in our schools: Dickinson, G.M. Hopkins, Langston Hughes, Melville, Thoreau, and so on. The crucial point in studying these authors' work from a gay perspective is not to claim them as homosexual, though better cases can be made on that point for some than others. The purpose in raising the possibility is to gain insight into the writing through hypothesis. We know that gay identity as we understand it today is not a trans-historic means of interpretation (Boswell 1992; Epstein 1987; Halperin 1990; Stein 1992). But the fact that a particular author might have experienced same-gender attraction and not have identified as gay in the modern sense should not prevent us from examining the importance of this attraction to his thinking and its *possible* influence on his work. For example, analysis of Thoreau's poem, "Sympathy" ("Lately, alas, I knew a gentle boy") is en-riched by considering its homoromanticism. Additionally, a hypothesis of Thoreau's homosexuality is an exciting criterion for probing the mindset of *Walden*. This exercise is intellectually satisfying, even if we cannot find explicit reference to gay self-awareness either in *Walden* itself or in the jour-nals (Harding 1991). As Eve Kosofsky Sedgwick has observed: "no one *can* know in *advance* where the limits of a gay-centered inquiry are to be drawn, or where a gay theorizing of and through even the hegemonic high culture of the Euro-American tradition may need or be able to lead" (Sedgwick 1990, emphasis hers).

Teachers have taught Willa Cather's "Paul's Case" without mention of the possible homosexuality, either of the character Paul or of the author. Though it may not be critical to know details about Cather's woman companions, un-derstanding "Paul's Case" is impoverished without a gay lens. Examination of Cather's early condemnation of Oscar Wilde brings even greater nuance to the analysis (Summers 1990).

A similar argument can be made for studying *Billy Budd* as a story of re-pressed homoerotic desire and its consequences. The insights gained there provide the means for a different understanding of *Moby Dick* or "Bartleby the Scrivener." Students could sample documentation of the passionate relationship between Melville and Hawthorne (Rowse 1977). These observations would be commonplace in some universities, but they would be extraordinary anywhere else. The routine unsensationalized inclusion of homosexual possibilities in the high school curriculum would have a profoundly positive effect.

Social Construction Theory

Social studies and literature units inevitably lead to the issue of social constructionism. This compelling nominalist theory, propounded by Foucault and others (Foucault 1978; McIntosh 1968; Weeks 1985), posits that categories of identity are completely a creation of culture. Society develops labels and social scripts for the creation of identities that are entirely arbitrary. Social constructionists believe that there are no essential, inborn, and ageless criteria for identity, but that certain human features assume importance as a result of society's temporal needs or dictates.

This theory has assumed a central place in modern discourse about sexuality, and one does not have to subscribe to its most extreme forms to recognize either its power or its appeal. Whatever the characteristic under consideration, whether sexuality, race, gender, or some other, a social constructionist analysis is a useful one. It is especially appealing to young people, for whom society's dictates are a locus both of self-reference and potential rebellion.

Although one may begin with sexuality, the implications of social constructionism are broad. Discussions of culturally imposed categories of sexual identity can lead to poignant conversations among groups of diverse high school students. In Cambridge they have struggled over what it means to be Jewish or black in America and what is essential to a woman's identity. One biracial student talked about her inability to choose between being black or white and her desire to be both and neither. She did not appear to be a pathetic lost soul, searching for meaning in her racial identity. She was a strong, self-respecting person, who expressed impatience with society's narrow categories and perhaps with any category based on pigmentation. Her need to be accepted just as herself was not surprising in a teenager, but her capacity to inspire others to challenge universally accepted racial dichotomies was extraordinary. As a child of mixed parentage, she had doubtless given much thought to the question. However, it was the social constructionist discussion, prompted by the issue of homosexuality, that gave her the incentive to speak out. Through her example, all students were challenged to examine the power of socially constructed labels to determine their lives. Indeed, gay and lesbian youth themselves, for all comforts to be found in the safe harbor of a gay identity, may be too trapped to some degree by the limits of its current definition (Sears 1990).

Staff Training

Any curricular reform is dependent to some degree on staff development. Inclusion of homosexuality is particularly so, from the standpoints of both methodology and content.

Preparing teachers just to broach the subject of homosexuality with their students is the first task. Teachers must work out their own feelings on the issue and then be trained to handle the discomfort of some students, as well as the inevitable "are you one of them" question. We assume that teachers eventually can learn to deal with this issue as they have learned to handle other controversial issues in the classroom. Still, a comfortable willingness on the part of teachers to include homosexuality in their curricula is not the last consideration.

Unlike many other subjects, the content of this area of study is markedly absent from teacher preparation syllabi. A small number of colleges today offer gay studies courses; a handful may integrate some gay material into broader courses. One has little assurance that incoming secondary school faculty have taken any of these. One can be certain that the vast majority of veteran faculty have had no formal training in gay studies, although they may have read something on their own. Most are dependent on the same sources that inform the general public. Such a superficial acquaintance with the subject is hardly reassuring.

But neither is teacher ignorance about homosexuality surprising. In the 1970s, when curricular diversity required the addition of African-American, Asian-American, or Hispanic-American materials, how many teachers or curriculum specialists were prepared for that task? Indeed, most at that time

A serious effort to include gay and lesbian curricula in high schools must entail comprehensive staff development.

required some compensatory education. Today teachers may have brought themselves up to speed on certain facets of multiculturalism; and universities are doing far more than they were 25 years ago to prepare beginning teachers for diversity. Nevertheless, as far as sexuality is concerned, the gap between the need and the preparation is still great.

A serious effort to include gay and lesbian curricula in high schools must entail comprehensive staff development, including both a general program in "gay sensitivity" and the imparting of substantive information about homosexuality and about gay history and culture. Good intentions are not enough. These programs are the responsibility of the secondary schools themselves and of the teacher training institutions.

If school personnel attempt to bring about change without proper training, there is great risk of failure. The least homophobic teacher may be incapable of answering accurately the most basic questions about homosexuality. It is arguably better not to bring up the subject at all than to repeat even well-intentioned stereotypes or disproven theories. Granted, teachers don't have to be omniscient; on the other hand, sexuality, like race, is one area in which a modicum of ignorance can cause great harm.

Similarly, a reluctant or unhappy teacher can be worse than no teacher at all. It would be a mistake at first to *require* all teachers to teach this subject, especially without proper training. Students are very good at detecting insincerity, and we don't want the message to be "I'm being forced to deal with this subject even though I am uncomfortable with it and don't approve of homosexuality."

All teachers, however, should be required to interrupt expressions of homophobia, if only as a violation of school rules. Even that minimal intervention requires some training. But if a teacher with such training is still uncomfortable with curriculum inclusion, it would be better to start with those who are willing. This should not be a top-down reform with mandated curricular change. It is preferable to inspire the changes with encouragement at the building level and the grassroots. Later, when a critical mass of support has been established among the faculty, further persuasion may be attempted. Even a partial transformation of the personnel and curriculum should have significant impact.

Age Appropriateness

Last, it is crucial that the curriculum be age appropriate. One may scratch one's head over the arbitrariness of grade level, but there should be no disagreement over gauging the content of the sexuality lesson to the sexual maturity of the student. *Heather Has Two Mommies* (Newman 1989) was written for the children of lesbians, not for a general children's audience. The book includes an explanation of alternative insemination and is not suitable for all young children. In fact, it was recommended as a teachers' resource in the Children of the Rainbow Curriculum and was not required for students.

That is not to say that there cannot be materials about gay parents that would be good for all young children. Such a book would describe gay family relationships in terms that a child would understand. It might even, despite the outcries over *Daddy's Roommate* (Willhoite 1990), include an illustration of two same-gender parents in a bed. The child would be expected to interpret the bedroom scene in the same way he understands the "heterosexual bedroom" as a place where mommy/daddy, daddy/girlfriend, or mommy/boyfriend sleep. As the student's sophistication about sexuality develops at home, in the community, and at school, the gay and lesbian curriculum should keep pace.

The Challenge

Teachers may be encouraged and supported in anti-homophobia work by the passage of legislation protecting gay/lesbian/bisexual youth from harassment and discrimination in schools. Teachers often need some form of official dictum to support them in a sensitive enterprise; they want to have a defense against attack from political foes or anxious parents. So far, however, anti-harassment law applicable to minors has not covered harassment based on sexual orientation. Moreover, "gay rights" laws do not apply to minors.

Even where policies protecting gay youth exist, they cannot be construed easily to call for curriculum. As we have seen in Massachusetts, protecting gay youth from assault or suicide and offering them counseling are seen as separate from presenting gay subject matter. The first three are defended as care-giving, an approved function of schools in the last thirty years; the last is condemned as proselytizing, teaching kids to be gay. One opponent of gay curriculum, the attorney for the New York school board that rejected the Rainbow, said in a radio debate with me ("Talk of the Nation," National Public Radio, 22 December 1992) that he approved of teaching about homosexuality in schools as long as it was presented alongside drug addiction, alcoholism, and other evils.

It will take great courage for schools to begin curricular inclusion of gay and lesbian materials. Such innovation may be supported in the end by two powerful arguments. First, we must hold to the fact that learning about gay life does not cause young people to become gay, though it might encourage those who are struggling with their homosexual desires to feel better about their gay identities. This coming to happier terms with one's sexuality must benefit the entire community, since we know the misery and harm that can come both to the gay person and his loved ones from repression and hiding. Second, we must maintain our professional integrity as teachers in our respective disciplines. We will not advance learning or model honesty if we persist in ignoring certain facts of history, science, or artistic representation which some faction or other may object to. That brand of political correctness, exercised by the majority, is as much a threat to the ideal of education as the more often decried tyranny of the left.

If anyone is recruited in this campaign to cast off one nature and assume another, let it be the bigot, who learns to accept this difference of sexual expression. As proof of that possibility I offer an examination excerpt written by a student at Cambridge Rindge and Latin School, in Cambridge, Massachusetts, in 1992. This student had previously done an oral class report on discrimination against gays, in which he admitted to being from a neighborhood in which gay-bashing was common and to having been a party to it. He wrote:

> One thing that changed me the most, and made me become a better person, and made me understand better, was the topic on homosexuals been discriminated against.
>
> People nowadays, a lot of people that I know, don't take this serious. They think it's a big joke to laugh about but in my opinion it is something we all women and men should work on to make people understand the effects of life, so we all could live hopefully forevermore.

I must admit myself. I used to hate even hearing the word homosexual. I used to think that they were not regular people, so they should all get eliminated from our society but now I have a different perspective. And because of the class and studying about this topic in particular changed a great deal. People should not be discriminated against no matter what. . .

References

Boswell, John. "Categories, Experience, and Sexuality." In *Forms of Desire: Sexual Orientation and the Social Constructionist Controversy*, edited by Edward Stein. New York: Routledge, 1992.

Cass, V.C. "Homosexual Identity Formation: Testing a Theoretical Model." *The Journal of Sex Research* 20 (1984).

Coleman, E. *Integrated Identity for Gays and Lesbians: Psychotherapeutic Approaches for Emotional Well-Being.* Binghampton, N.Y.: Harrington Park Press, 1988.

Donnerstein, E., et al. "Estimating Community Standards: The Use of Social Science Evidence in an Obscenity Prosecution." *Public Opinion Quarterly* 55 (Spring 1993): 1.

Epstein, Steven. "Gay Politics, Ethnic Identity: The Limits of Social Constructionism." *Socialist Review* (May-August 1987).

Ferreira, A., et al. "The Contributions of Lesbian and Gay Teachers." Panel at the third annual conference of the Gay and Lesbian School Teachers Network, Milton Academy, Milton, Mass., 1 March 1993.

Foucault, Michel. *The History of Sexuality. Volume 1: An Introduction.* Robert Hurley, trans. New York: Pantheon, 1978.

Gonsiorek, John C. "Mental Health Issues of Gay and Lesbian Adolescents." *Journal of Adolescent Health Care* 9 (1988): 114-22.

The Governor's Commission on Gay and Lesbian Youth. *Making Schools Safe for Gay and Lesbian Youth: Education Report.* Boston: Commonwealth of Massachusetts, 25 February 1993.

Haignere, C.S. "Planned Parenthood Harris Poll Findings: Teens' Sexuality Knowledge and Beliefs." Paper presented at the Annual Children's' Defense Fund National Conference, Washington, D.C., 1987.

Halperin, David. *One Hundred Years of Homosexuality.* New York: Routledge, 1990.

Harding, Walter. "Thoreau's Sexuality." *Journal of Homosexuality* 21, no. 3 (1991).

Herdt, Gilbert, ed. *Gay and Lesbian Youth.* Binghampton, N.Y.: Harrington Park Press, 1989.

Herdt, Gilbert, and Boxer, Andrew. *Children of Horizons: How Gay and Lesbian Teens Are Leading a New Way Out of the Closet.* Boston: Beacon Press, 1993.

Herek, G., and Berill, K. *Hate Crimes: Confronting Violence Against Lesbians and Gay Men.* Newbury Park, Calif.: Sage, 1992.

Hetrick, Emery S., and Martin, A. Damien. "Developmental Issues and Their Resolution for Gay and Lesbian Adolescents." *Journal of Homosexuality* 14, nos. 1 and 2 (1987).

Hetrick, Emery S., and Martin, A. Damien. "The Stigmatization of the Gay and Lesbian Adolescent." *Journal of Homosexuality* 15, nos. 1 and 2 (1988).

Hunter, Joyce, and Schaecher, Robert. "Stresses on Lesbian and Gay Adolescents in Schools." *Work in Education* (Spring 1987).

Kirk, Marshall, and Madsen, Hunter. *After the Ball: How America Will Conquer Its Fear and Hatred of Gays in the 90's.* New York: Doubleday, 1989.

Levin, J., and McDevitt, J. *Hate Crimes: The Rising Tide of Bigotry and Bloodshed.* New York: Plenum, 1993.

Licata, Salvatore. "The Homosexual Rights Movement in the U.S.: A Traditionally Over-looked Area of American History." *Journal of Homosexuality* 6, nos. 1-2 (1980-81).

McIntosh, Mary. "The Homosexual Role." *Social Problems* 16 (1968).

McManus, M., et al. *Oregon's Sexual Minority Youth: An At-Risk Population. Lesbian, Gay and Bisexual Youth.* Portland, Oregon: Task Force on Sexual Minority Youth, 1991.

Newman, Leslea. *Heather Has Two Mommies.* Boston: Alyson, 1989.

Remafedi, Gary. "Homosexual Youth: A Challenge to Contemporary Society." *JAMA* 258 (10 July 1987).

Remafedi, Gary. "Fundamental Issues in the Care of Homosexual Youth." *Medical Clinics of North America* 74 (September 1990).

Rowse, A.L. *Homosexuals in History: A Study of Ambivalence in Society, Literature and the Arts.* New York: Dorset, 1977.

Savin-Williams, R.C. *Gay and Lesbian Youth: Expressions of Identity.* Bristol, Pa.: Hemisphere Publishing, 1990.

Schoenhals, Martin. *Youth Survey Report.* Philadelphia Lesbian and Gay Task Force, 1992.

Sears, James T. *Growing Up Gay in the South.* Binghampton, N.Y.: Haworth, 1990.

Seattle Commission on Children and Youth. *Report on Gay and Lesbian Youth in Seattle.* 1988.

Sedgwick, Eve Kosofsky. "Pedagogy in the Context of an Antihomophobic Project." *South Atlantic Quarterly* 89, no. 1 (1990).

Stafford, J. Martin. "In Defense of Gay Lessons" *Journal of Moral Education* 17 (1988).

Stein, Edward. "Introduction." In *Forms of Desire: Sexual Orientation and the Social Con-structionist Controversy*, edited by Edward Stein. New York: Routledge, 1992.

Summers, Claude J. *Gay Fictions: Wilde to Stonewall: Studies in a Male Homosexual Lit-erary Tradition.* New York: Continuum, 1990.

Troiden, R.R. *Gay and Lesbian Identity: A Sociological Analysis.* Dix Hills, N.Y.: General Hall, 1988.

U.S. Dept. of Health and Human Services. *Report of the Secretary's Task Force on Youth Suicide.* Washington, D.C.: U.S. Government Printing Office, 1989.

Weeks, Jeffrey. *Sexuality and Its Discontents: Meanings, Myths, and Modern Sexuality.* London: Routledge and Kegan Paul, 1985.

Weinberg, T.S. *Gay Men, Gay Selves.* New York: Irvington, 1983.

Willhoite, Michael. *Daddy's Roommate.* Boston: Alyson, 1990.

Zelnik, M., and Shah, F.K. "First Intercourse Among Young Americans." *Family Planning Perspectives* 15 (1983).

Self-Censorship of Picture Books About Gay and Lesbian Families*

by John Warren Stewig

The rapidly changing roles of lesbians and gay males in American society has evoked contentious debate. The talk is everywhere. As Sullivan (1993) points out: "In place of the silence that once encased the lives of homosexuals, there is now a loud argument. And there is no easy going back" (p. 24). Intensified by the debate over gays in the military (Browning 1993), fueled by increasing numbers of scientific reports about the biological bases of homosexuality (Burr 1993), and by concerns over the related illness, AIDS (Weiss 1993), this debate has permeated public discourse. As Kopkind (1993) says: "The gay movement is unavoidable. It fills the media, charges politics, saturates popular and elite culture" (p. 577).

Contention about this has reached even the ordinarily more tranquil backwater of public education, as exemplified in the forced ouster of New York City public schools chancellor, Joseph Fernandez, over his proposed "Rainbow Curriculum," designed to help children understand the diversity present in America. This attempt to control the ideas children encounter in schools is common today.

For example, censorship is currently one of the most *au courant* of topics. Efforts to ban books increase. Professional journals regularly feature articles

*An earlier version of this essay was published in *The New Advocate* 7 (Summer 1994): 184-92.

about it (Loch-Wouters 1991). Convention sessions on the topic attract wide audiences. Professional organizations devote staff time to combat increasing efforts to remove books from library shelves. All this attention to the problem of censorship is indeed commendable.

But another equally important problem needs attention: the problem of those books that never make it to the shelves in the first place (Harmon 1987; Woods and Perry-Holmes 1982). As the submerged part of an iceberg is always bigger than the visible tip, so there's a much larger invisible problem floating beneath the surface of visible censorship. That is the process of teachers and librarians not buying a book because it may cause trouble in the school. And at what cost to child readers' curiosity about the world do we make such decisions?

School libraries now include books about death, divorce, drugs, and suicide. Authors write, publishers produce, and librarians purchase books about these topics. In addition, the majority of both school and public librarians conscientiously search for positive reviews of, and then order, books representing ethnic minorities.

But teachers and librarians probably overlook another largely invisible minority. What sort of representation of the American family is found in the books on our shelves? For more than a decade, sociologists have been telling us that families no longer are made up primarily of a husband, wife, and that statistical 2.5 children. Families are, indeed, an increasingly more diverse array of adult and child combinations. Yet what kinds of families do the books in school classrooms and library collections show? Do they in fact show that increasing numbers of children are parented by lesbians and gay males? Increasing numbers of these men and women are choosing to take more active roles in parenting their own, or their partner's, children. In fact, Patterson (1992) reports that estimates of the number of children being raised by such parents ranges from 6 million to 14 million. Books that depict such family structures are being published and should be accessible to young readers.

In this essay I describe three such books, identifying their strengths and weaknesses. I suggest that teachers must seek out this type of book and then advocate that libraries purchase them. The sample discussed is limited to three books because they are among the very few picture book fiction titles available that deal with children in families headed by lesbians and gays. Publishers have done more on this topic for older readers in both fiction and

Books that depict [gay- and lesbian- parented] family structures are being published and should be accessible to young readers.

information books (Drescher 1980; Tax 1981). But picture books on the topic are equally critical, so that young children can see the diversity that the word *family* conveys today.

To begin, let us consider *Heather Has Two Mommies* by Leslea Newman, about a young girl living with two lesbians (Newman 1989). As Barbara Grier, vice president of Naiad Press, points out:

> In our society, women are socialized to marry and have a family. As a result, there's an inordinate number of lesbians who have children. And I know literally hundreds of lesbians who have chosen to have babies. (James 1991, pp. D1-2).

After introducing the main character, Heather, the author in a brief flashback describes how this family was formed. The details of the artificial insemination of Heather's biological mother, Jane, are given clearly, and that may bother some readers. However, the emphasis throughout the book is on the love the two women feel for each other and for their child. Much of the book focuses on the everyday details of three-year-old Heather's life: picnicking with her family, doing different activities with each of her mommies, and going to playgroup.

While at playgroup, Heather becomes aware that she is the only child there who has two mommies. But she also discovers that one of the children has only a mother and a sister, another has two fathers (his stepdaddy and his biological father), and yet another has two daddies who live together, apparently in a gay male relationship, although that is not stated. In short, what Heather's teacher helps the children understand, using a book about families and a follow-up drawing activity, is that families come in all kinds of variations.

In places some of the writing seems a bit forced; that David's siblings are all adopted is natural enough, but that one of them is in a wheelchair seems a bit gratuitous. This small caveat aside, the book presents a naturalistic examination of a day in the life of a preschooler living in a family representative of the family variety in America today. As the reviewer for the February 1990 *Bulletin of the Center for Children's Books* noted, "This is a positive, if idealized, portrait of a loving lesbian family, and it preaches a respect for all kinds of families" (p. 144). Such reviews are more helpful, because they

73

evaluate the book, rather than simply describe its plot, as did the review in *Small Press Book Review.* The black and white pencil illustrations in a flat and patterned style are augmented at one place by drawings of their families ostensibly done by the children themselves.

Michael Willhoite's book, *Daddy's Roommate* (1990), is a large (8½" x 11") format, which presents well the author's cartoon-like, full-color illustrations. The unnamed young male narrator is older than Heather, although the text here is simpler, for the most part a single line of words set beneath the full-page pictures. Like the other book, this is primarily a pleasantly innocuous account of the young boy's life. First he describes the things that his daddy and the roommate do, all of which seem commonplace. For example, the page that describes "working together" shows one of the men vacuuming and the other dusting. A following section shows activities that the boy does with Frank, the roommate, such as telling each other jokes and riddles, catching bugs for show-and-tell, and reading. In what is evidently a joint-custody arrangement, the child lives with his mother during the week, but on weekends enjoys doing such things as going to ball games and working in the yard with the two men.

Like the book about Heather, this story minimizes any problems these living arrangements may occasion. The young narrator here says, "My Mommy and Daddy got a divorce last year," but there's no reaction to that statement. The book briefly alludes to the normal disagreements that plague any couple. For example, talking of the two men, the narrator says they "sometimes even fight together, but they always make up." At the end, the narrator asks his mother what it means to be gay. She replies that being gay is "just one more kind of love." Because his daddy and Frank are happy, the child is happy, too. This may be, as one critic has pointed out,

> A little rosy perhaps — the mother, for example, seems miraculously devoid of bitterness. But then, this is a children's book, meant to make a point without hitting kids over the head. (James 1991, pp. D1-2)

Another reviewer, in the 1 March 1991 issue of *Booklist*, agreed that this is "an upbeat, positive portrayal of a situation common to many children with gay fathers" (p. 1403). The review in the 7 December 1990 issue of *Publishers*

Weekly commented on the "suitably straightforward" text and declared the format of single lines of copy underneath full-page illustrations to be "easily accessible to the intended audience" (p. 80). In closing, the reviewer commented on the "stabilizing air of warmth and familiarity in the book" (p. 80). In a gay periodical, *The Advocate* (1 January 1991), the reviewer commented that: "The message, supported by bright, expressive art [is] sure to catch the attention of the under-5 crowd" (p. 71).

Despite these positive reviews, many librarians probably chose not to purchase the book. According to an article in the April 1995 *American Libraries*, *Daddy's Roommate* was the year's "most challenged" book.

The oldest of the three books, *Jenny Lives with Eric and Martin* (Bosche 1983), originally was published in Denmark in 1981, then republished in Great Britain and made available by an American distributor. It also is the only book illustrated with black-and-white photographs, rather than with artist's illustrations. This confronts more directly the problems people with traditional values may have in dealing with this sort of living arrangement. Much of the book is a pleasant account of the daily activities of five-year-old Jenny. She and the men enjoy an ice cream bar sitting in the sun on the step outside their house, fix a small hole in her bicycle tire, and play lotto on a quiet Saturday evening. The book touches on the minor disagreements that surface in any family: Martin and Eric squabble over whose turn it is to cook one evening.

A more unpleasant encounter occurs when the three inadvertently bump into a neighbor, Mrs. Andrews, on the sidewalk. Though the men apologize, she is not mollified and says unpleasant things to them, which Jenny does not understand. Eric explains:

> "We call it that [gay] when two men love each other and live together like Martin and I do," says Eric. . . . "There are some people who can't understand it. They think it is strange for two men to live together, because it isn't very common. Perhaps someone has told them it is wrong. So they get scared or angry. It is often like that when people can't understand something." (p. 50)

Jenny and the men work through her confusion and fear by drawing some pictures about the event and a happy resolution to this cartoon encounter,

They show child readers, no matter what their own family structure is, that families are as richly diverse as the people who make them up.

which mirrors their own situation. This conclusion, plus a short ending scene with her friend Danny, will seem a bit unrealistic to adults, but together they serve a cathartic purpose for young Jenny.

The review in a British publication, *The School Librarian* (September 1984), commended the book, admitting that it would be "controversial, of course," but went on to ask: "Do we want children to go on believing that gay men are all freaks, dangerous, and probably criminal?" Admitting that books that set out to dispel a harmful myth are suspect, the review comments that children will probably be "sufficiently intrigued by the photographs to want to read the text." The book offers librarians and teachers the opportunity to "explain that it is wrong to assume that everyone is heterosexual. . . . Why shouldn't children know that?"

A British reviewer (1984), Peggy Heeks, commended the "matter-of-fact" text about this "charming five year old." Heeks did comment that "If we turn to the child's viewpoint, there is an obvious value to those living in such households in having a book which reflects their circumstances." She raises a literary question, however, in commenting:

> It is significant that when the author wishes to set out the moral issues raised by this family group, she has to do so in a little homily in cartoon form, outside the main framework of the text. Almost inevitably, the explanation becomes less than honest, and many major points are avoided altogether. (p. 27)

An American specialty periodical, *New Directions for Women* (July 1984), also reviewed the book, commenting positively on the way the author presents "the texture of their lives through an ordinary weekend's events," and concludes that the book provides children with "a valuable and sensitive lesson in human relations" (p. 11). Another American specialty periodical, *Interracial Books for Children Bulletin* (1984) commented that the book "deals honestly with gay relationships" and, because of this, declared it to be "a necessity. . . well worth purchasing" (p. 16).

These three books are examples of what can be done for young readers to help them understand that the word *family* can mean many different kinds of living arrangements when the people involved in them care genuinely about each other. In each book we have a young child living in such an arrange-ment, understanding it with the help of those adults involved, and for the most part going about the daily business of living.

Are the books fine literature, or are they merely useful? Each would in-deed be a better book if the text flowed more smoothly, if a talented editor had helped the authors smooth over some of the awkwardness that at times surfaces in the words. Similarly, the illustrations in all three could be more professionally done. None has the polished visual panache we have come to expect in picture books from major publishers. While we do not set aside our concerns about literary quality, we do remain aware that the first books to deal with any topic are often less well-crafted than later books. For exam-ple, the first books on premarital pregnancy were considerably less effective than books that followed. We have to support writers dealing with topics new to children's literature, knowing that more skillful works will follow. The topic of lesbians and gays is one that no major publisher has as yet been will-ing to approach in picture book format. Until mainstream publishers are willing to produce such books, we must support the small press publishers with the courage to do so.

Nonetheless, the books present an aspect of our real world today. They show child readers, no matter what their own family structure is, that fami-lies are as richly diverse as the people who make them up. Such books as these deserve a place in library collections, where, of course, we do not want to represent the world only as it was several decades ago or as it is idealized.

The issue of self-censorship is far broader than the particulars of the rep-resentation of lesbian and gay male parents in books. Censorship concerns intellectual curiosity. Do we really want to encourage children to wonder about their world? Do we value children asking questions about topics that interest them, or do we want only the inquiry with which we, as adults, are comfortable?

To the degree that self-censorship exists, we are building libraries and book collections that make adults comfortable, not necessarily ones that will serve as places where children can explore the world that surrounds them. Blocking out certain topics, such as sexual orientation, only convinces children that schools are not important places to learn, perhaps even that "books them-selves will seem obsolete to them" (Varlejs 1986, p. 84).

[Books about gay male and lesbian families] are important for children growing up in a lesbian or gay male family. They are equally important for children growing up in heterosexual families . . .

In a country and a generation in which two-thirds of all first marriages end in divorce (White 1990), more and more children are living in a wider variety of formed and re-formed families. Some children are themselves growing up in a lesbian or gay male family. For these children, it is as important an affirmation that they see themselves in books as it is important that ethnic minority children seen themselves in books. This is critical, even when some parents object to such books. For we must, as William E. Sheerin has said, balance the "interests of the community" with the "rights of the individual" (1991, p. 442). Certainly schools respect individual parents' rights to make decisions about what their own children may read, but such choices cannot be allowed to limit what other children may learn from books. Teachers must take the responsibility to make available for children books that represent the whole range of our world today, even when some of the topics may make some of us personally uncomfortable.

Community interests are served when teachers know about the available books and add them to school classroom and library collections. It is difficult to learn about these books though reviews, however. *Book Review Index* reports that only three major publishers of reviews chose to review any of these books. One British library publication reviewed one of the books. And one British and one American newspaper reviewed the books. Three limited-circulation, special interest periodicals each reviewed one of the books. If reviewers working with major journals in this country were asked why the books were not reviewed, most undoubtedly would point to the limited number of reviews they have space to publish and perhaps to their reservations about the literary qualities of these works.

This is an interesting, marked contrast to the circumstances surrounding the reviewing of books on other topics. Take, for example, the case of *I Have a Sister, My Sister Is Deaf* by Jeanne Peterson (1977), a book about deafness that seems mawkish at best. It is written in pseudo-first-person narration, quite unrelated to the way real children talk. Despite this, the book, on a topic librarians are careful to include in collections, was reviewed by no less than 14 reviewing sources. Of the three books considered here, one was reviewed by four sources, and the other two by fewer than that. Clearly, finding reliable critical analysis about these books will be a significant problem.

Many schools probably did not purchase these books because they were reviewed infrequently. Unfortunately, by now many librarians have heard about the books through the wide publicity given to post-purchase censorship efforts, notably as reported in a continuing series of letters last year to the editor of *American Libraries*. Such efforts undoubtedly will make publishers more reluctant to publish, and librarians more reluctant to purchase, such titles. This makes teacher support all the more critical. It also means that curriculum supervisors and school boards must support including such books in school libraries.

Such books as these, and others that need to be published on this topic, are important for children growing up in a lesbian or gay male family. They are equally important for children growing up in heterosexual families, for seeing such diversity in books can help all children more accurately understand the variety of life today.

For teachers who are committed to making schools a safe place to learn about the world in all its variations, the tasks are clear. First, we need to search out reviews of such books, and this means reading other than the two or three best-known reviewing journals, identified by Crow (1986). Second, we need to take energetic action to seek out the catalogues of small presses, which currently are more likely to publish such books than are major publishers. Horning (1993) has compiled a useful source of information about such presses. Third, we need to urge librarians to consider those books on an individual basis, not simply deciding *a priori* because of the topic to exercise self-censorship. By supporting librarians in adding such books to collections, we send an important message to mainstream publishers: We want this sort of material to be available.

References

Bosche, S. *Jenny Lives with Eric and Martin*. London: GMP, 1983.

Browning, F. "Boys in the Barracks." *Mother Jones* 18, no. 2 (1993): 24-25.

Burr, C. "Homosexuality and Biology." *The Atlantic Monthly* (March 1993): pp. 47-65.

Crow, S.R. "The Reviewing of Controversial Juvenile Books: A Study." *School Library Media Quarterly* 13, no. 14 (1986): 83-86.

Drescher, J. *Your Family, My Family*. New York: Walker, 1980.

Harmon, C. "Multicultural/Nonsexist Collections: A Closer Look." *Top of the News* 43, no. 3 (1987): 303-306.

Heeks, P. "A Family Affair." *Times Education Supplement*, 13 January 1984, p. 27.

Horning, K.T. *Alternative Press Publishers of Children's Books: A Directory*. Madison, Wis.: Cooperative Children's Book Center, 1993.

James, S. "When Mommy (or Daddy) Is Gay." *St. Petersburg Times*, 2 January 1991, pp. D1-D2.

Kopkind, A. "The Gay Movement." *The Nation*, 3 May 1993, pp. 577, 590-602.

Loch-Wouters, M. "Begin2

ner's Luck Has Just Run Out." *Journal of Youth Services in Libraries* 4, no. 3 (1991): 261-65.

Newman, L. *Heather Has Two Mommies*. Boston: Alyson, 1989.

Patterson, C.J. "Children of Gay and Lesbian Parents." *Child Development* 63 (1992): 1025-42.

Peterson, J. *I Have a Sister, My Sister Is Deaf*. New York: Harper & Row, 1977.

Sheerin, W.E. "Absolutism on Access and Confidentiality: Principled or Irresponsible?" *American Libraries* 22, no. 5 (1991): 442.

Sullivan, A. "The Politics of Homosexuality." *The New Republic*, 10 May 1993, pp. 24-26.

Tax, M. *Families*. Boston: Little, Brown, 1981.

Varlejs, J., ed. *Freedom of Information and Youth*. Jefferson, N.C.: McFarland, 1986.

Weiss, R.A. "How Does HIV Cause AIDS?" *Science*, 28 May 1993, pp. 1273-79.

White, L.K. "Determinants of Divorce." *Journal of Marriage and the Family* 52 (1990): 904-12.

Willhoite, M. *Daddy's Roommate*. Boston: Alyson, 1990.

Woods, L.B., and Perry-Holmes, C. "The Flak if We Had *The Joy of Sex* Here." *Library Journal* 107 (1982): 1711-15.

Bringing Gay and Lesbian Literature Out of the Closet*

by Vicky Greenbaum

When a student at the high school where I once taught decided to come out as a lesbian in front of the whole school at a campus meeting, she told a story about her Spanish class. In class one day, her teacher told students to describe in Spanish their ideal love, using correct pronouns and other grammatical tools. Boys were to describe their ideal woman, girls were to describe their ideal man. The young lesbian told her campus audience how she sat, brow in a knot, afraid that students might be asked to read their descriptions out loud. She didn't want to give in to the assignment's implicit heterosexism, but writing about a woman would have meant a surprise revelation about herself to the class. Finally, she decided to write the assignment without reference to gender. Standing in front of the campus meeting, this lesbian student said, "I'm tired of everyone assuming that I'm straight."

Unfortunately, in less hospitable surroundings, where people are penalized for not being straight, gay and lesbian students often have wished, for their own safety, to be assumed heterosexual. While I, as an openly lesbian faculty member, teach that being open about sexuality is a right instead of a

*An earlier, brief version of this essay was published as "Literature Out of the Closet: Bringing Gay and Lesbian Texts and Subtexts Out in High School English," *English Journal* (September 1994): 71-74.

privilege, I also explain the long history of hiding that is most obvious in the literature taught in English classes. Any hint of homosexuality is suppressed when discussing texts in most classrooms, yet heterosexual content is acknowledged if not thoroughly explored. What students need now, I believe, is a balanced view of literature: Gay and lesbian students need to know that voices like theirs are active, and straight-identified students need to see that there are many ways to be sexual in the world. This means that all students should be made aware of homoerotic subtexts in literature of the past and of gay and lesbian voices in more recent literature.

Emily Dickinson's letters to the Rev. Wadsworth and Mr. Higginson are often mentioned in English classes; her loving letters to Susan Gilbert Dickinson are not. Shakespeare's bawdy heterosexual double-entendres rate a mention; his love sonnets to several British noblemen do not. When teaching Tennessee Williams' *Cat on a Hot Tin Roof*, teachers mention the strong female characterization of Maggie, along with her passionate desire to bear Brick a child; but they usually ignore the agony of Brick's self-inflicted homophobia. Alice Walker's *The Color Purple* is taught with increasing frequency as a brilliant novel about black life; the lesbian relationship that thrives at the novel's center goes unmentioned.

Too often, current teaching of literature in American classrooms tends to assume that lesbian and gay content is not there, that lesbian and gay students do not exist, and that lesbian and gay experience is invisible. Because of the conventions of morality, often explicitly homophobic, the pervading assumption remains that upset the lesbian student: every text, and every person, is assumed to be straight. Correcting this error is a matter of conscious awareness. Because exclusion and fear create pain and distance for students, teachers must ensure that gay and lesbian voices are heard. Invisibility and silence hurt gay and lesbian people.

As this realization dawned for me, I began cautiously to teach gay subtexts in literature in my public-school English classrooms eight years ago. As a then-closeted lesbian teacher, I felt the risks most keenly. Therefore, I developed some ground rules for myself:

- Always mention all the subtexts, not just homoerotic ones. Be aware of race, sex, and cultural differences, too, so that all students can begin noticing subtexts on their own.

> *My first impulse, as a closeted teacher, was to run and hide behind the nearest potted palm.*

- If possible, wait until trust is established before working with difficult matters.
- Always be prepared for what might come up.

The results continued to be positive, in class after class, year after year. Entire classes began to notice often-ignored (or tiptoed-around) moments, such as Holden's visit to Mr. Antonelli's house in *Catcher in the Rye*, or the possibility that Tom in *The Glass Menagerie* might be gay. Although I did feel an inner tension, arising from my closeted discomfort, whenever homosexuality came out in a text, I noticed that my students' increasing comfort level eased my own inner strain. Indeed, by the time I'd switched coasts, becoming a (still-closeted) teacher on split English/Music assignment in an East Coast prep school, the discomfort was reduced to a small hardness in my midriff. After all, by January my ninth-grade English students were discovering homoerotic subtexts in *Julius Caesar* on their own.

A chance encounter with Steven, a member of the first senior English class I ever taught, gave me my first glimpse of how important this kind of understanding was for gay students. One weekend in April 1985, I attended a dance for gays and lesbians at the nearby university. Early in the evening, as I was dancing with my girlfriend in the very center of the not-yet-crowded dance floor, I saw Steven come in the door. He was holding hands with a taller, older, college man. Frozen with shock, I stopped dancing. My first impulse, as a closeted teacher, was to run and hide behind the nearest potted palm. But Steven beat me to it. As soon as I'd noticed him, he saw me, too; and he vanished behind the largest of the greens, dragging his friend behind him.

Suddenly I grinned, understanding his fear even as I realized that we were adrift in the same boat. We were both on homosexual territory with same-sex partners.

Eventually Steven must have made the same discovery, because I had barely explained the situation to my dance partner when Steven appeared at my elbow. "Hi, Ms. Greenbaum," he smiled sheepishly. After introducing our partners, we headed for the bar to grab a Calistoga and talk. He was clearly elated to be talking to me about being gay. At the end of the dance he said merrily, "See you in class!" and from then on, when I approached the classroom bungalow each day after lunch, Steven was there waiting.

He needed to talk about the fear of discovery, especially by his parents. He'd been sneaking down to the local gay bar for two years, meeting guys, making up stories to hide from parental scrutiny. Most of all, he was ready to learn more about the thoughtful side of being gay — "the mental side," he called it. His new college boyfriend was the first man with whom he had talked about books and gay culture.

One day, a new lightbulb went on over Steven's head. In the five remaining minutes of lunch period that day, he explained his idea. Our latest reading project was *The Secret Sharer* by Joseph Conrad, and the class was to have completed the novella for homework. "I think *Secret Sharer* is about being gay," Steven confided. "That's a good thesis," I agreed, and then we discussed Conrad's description of doubleness, secrecy, the men leaning together over a bed, and the sense of longing, imbued with silence and concealment, of two men together.

Over the next few lunch times, I met Steven for mini-seminars as he compiled evidence from the text in support of his idea. The need to keep homoeroticism hidden and subtextual in his own life lent flavor to his analysis of the literary subtext as an undercurrent, a hint of meaning not spelled out in the story. When students were discussing their writing assignment for the novella, Steven managed to bring up this idea in class. He felt the need to ask the question in homophobic disguise: "Is this about faggots?" I was able to frame a dignified reply, despite the irony: the first homophobic statement heard in class that year emanated from the mouth of this closeted teen. However, his paper on subtle homoeroticism merited an A; and as we adjourned for summer vacation, Steven requested a list of literature with gay subtexts. His excitement taught me that this invisible hunger might lurk everywhere, and it was time for me to think of strategies for feeding students something new and needed.

A few colleagues have reacted dismissively to what they call "fishing for extraneous debris" in literature. My response is that what the narrow eye views as "debris" is, in fact, central to many human lives. I challenge these colleagues to broaden their vision to include others beside themselves, beside the traditional Everyman that has dominated literary vision and practice for far too long. We can see the world as a bigger place now. As readers and teachers, we can know that the fear of displacement comes from the fallacy of one center. Instead, why not view life as a palette, or spectrum, of options? We can see that texts are written by people with personal lives, and that subtexts exist everywhere. This kind of vision is coming out even more as more gay and lesbian people come out in schools.

When I was able to safely come out, first in the intellectual openness of Phillips Academy's Andover Summer Session and then in the warmly openminded atmosphere of Northfield Mt. Hermon School, I found myself able to teach gay and lesbian literature as well. Midway through a summer literature class at Andover, I introduced *The Color Purple* as (among other things) a lesbian novel. My class read the novel, made maps of who was at the center of the book, discussed the absence of white people and the scarcity of men. We used *Purple* as a way to examine how literature works in society. Students read from their response logs and discussion ensued. I did not have to lead very much. Students invented dialogues between characters to explore feelings further. One exercise had students writing and acting out a dialogue between Celie and her "father." Students explored their feelings about lesbianism, from "eeew" to acceptance.

Not everyone is ready to emerge gleefully from the closet, ready to change the world.

My open lesbianism caused students to be gentler in expressing their homophobia than had I been seen as straight. One boy wrote, "It must be hard for you to hear people say 'Eeew' about you, so I'm sorry that was my first reaction." I encouraged them to explore the roots of "eeew," to see where such reactions come from, to see if they wanted to keep reacting that way. "Not if it hurts someone," a girl replied. Because the students saw me as a person they didn't want to hurt, and because Celie was a character with whom they were fully sympathetic, they were able to think openly about lesbian sexuality in writing and in life.

Another successful classroom experience involved a group of short stories: "So's Yo Mama" from Julie Blackwomon's collection in *Voyages Out 2* (published by Seal Press), "When You Grow to Adultery" from *Family Dancing* by David Leavitt, and "A Birthday Remembered" by Ann Allen Shockley, in *Between Mothers and Daughters* (Koppelman 1985). Students wrote and talked about what it might be like to have a lesbian mom (in the Blackwomon story) and to have lesbian and gay relatives or to be a homosexual relative (the Shockley and Leavitt pieces, respectively). We began with stories of relatives belonging to students, writing about a memorable (or difficult) experience or discovery about them. Then we read the stories, and students were ready to see how homosexual people can and do fit within family dynamics, which often are deeply complex themselves. This reading works best in the context of a unit of reading and thinking about families of all kinds.

Looking back, I think my most memorable teaching experiment happened when I taught Tennessee Williams' *Cat on a Hot Tin Roof* to summer school students in San Francisco. These students enrolled in my independent school literature class because they had failed their sophomore English classes in public high school, or because they were recent immigrants who were catching up on high school credits in order to graduate by the time they were 18. By the fifth week of our eight-week session, the students enjoyed my class, were used to writing daily, and felt at home in our discussions. We read *Cat* aloud, taking turns playing the parts, because Francisco's severe dyslexia prevented him from reading longer works at home and Yifang's English was still dependent on the translating services of his classroom neighbor Wu. After three days we were finished with reading the play, and I asked for the usual five questions as homework. Students knew to bring in questions to which they did not know the answers, interpretive questions as well as factual questions.

Tony, from a severe boys-only Catholic school, asked, "Why is Brick making a big deal about the handshake with his dead friend?" Tanisha, who had missed most of spring semester when she and her mom left her abusive stepfather to live in a women's shelter, had one answer, "Because he killed himself as a result, and Brick thinks he mistook himself for gay." Francisco, whose listening skills were sharp, gave a different answer, quoting Big Daddy when he says that love is love and nothing to be ashamed of. "So maybe he was gay?" I asked. Some students did not like this, thinking it perverted, weird, "eeew." I stirred the pot a little, mentioning for the first time that I am a lesbian. This created a sidebar of discussion, lasting perhaps 20 minutes, before I steered us back to the text. (Fortunately these summer sessions lasted three hours each morning.)

By the time we got to writing, students had thoroughly discussed sexuality in terms of the play, in terms of a real person (me), and in terms of people they knew and saw on the street. We also discussed Maggie's strength;

Why not banish fear and broaden the spectrum?

Brick's alcoholism; how families in the South differ from, or resemble, our own families; and how the dramatic structure of the play works. And so we wrote. The students could choose between a personal essay and an interpretive thesis. I wrote along with them. After a half hour, we would do some critiquing in small groups, then take the rest home to complete and polish toward a final draft.

The next day, we read the papers aloud and discussed some ideas. Yifang asked why a writer would choose a difficult and taboo subject like this one, and is it just an American thing? No one had an answer; and so after a few moments, I responded, mentioning Japanese author Yukio Mishima's gay novel, *Confessions of a Mask*, and André Gide's novels about French gay subculture. I also mentioned that Williams was gay.

Tony wondered why the teacher didn't tell him this when teaching *The Glass Menagerie* last year, and we discussed why authors' lives might or might not be important for readers to know about. Jennifer (one of two white people in the class, and one of two females as well) pointed out that heterosexuality gets talked about all the time, as with Maggie and Brick's marriage, so we may as well speak of other kinds of sexuality as well.

Finally, Marco (a recent, straight immigrant from Brazil who managed to convince homophobic Tony that not all gay guys want to "hit on" him the moment they see him) asked if that day's writing could be a story about what Williams was thinking when he wrote this play. After some discussion, the whole class accepted this, and the writing began.

Even without the luxury of a three-hour class, I want to repeat this kind of adventure in current classrooms. A little tinkering with focus, timing, and assignments is easily done. Because I like to allow my students to share in shaping our classwork, no two experiences are likely to be the same. We are not bored, and we are always wondering what we will discover next.

Stories of such discoveries abound. One kind of discovery that is always lurking behind the teaching experience is a new possibility about one's own sexuality. A colleague at a certain school (both place and person must remain nameless) experienced a kind of negative epiphany about her sexuality one morning when she was listening to a group of gay students come out in the school's public forum. The teacher whose epiphany I describe was a good teacher, in her first year at the school where she taught; and everyone expected her to remain on the faculty. Sitting in her school meeting, listening to the students come out, this teacher felt a terrible pressure building inside: How could she remain closeted in the face of such idealism, be it naive or courageous? She had heard the straight faculty at her lunch table speculating about what might happen to the students on the podium if they came out — there was talk of hockey sticks and assault in male dorms at night, of name calling and subtle attacks that might ensue. The closeted teacher remained silent during these lunch-time discussions, preferring to turn the conversation to her team rankings or to a new way of presenting a Shakespeare play to her sixth-period class.

After the school meeting, though, she heard people congratulating the openly gay students; negative comments may have been made sotto-voce in certain places, but she did not hear very many of those. Throughout the term, she worried: Should I come out? How can I? As she stood in her English class, teaching the use of transitions in essays, she felt her face color deeply as a student wondered how to make a link between a paragraph about gay students and another about his own homophobic self. He was watching her closely, she felt, measuring the quality of her response. Fighting to keep her voice noncommittal, she stuck closely to the mechanics of crafting an essay.

In the middle of teaching *Catcher in the Rye*, a girl posed questions about Mr. Antonelli being stereotypical in his gesture of reaching out to Holden as he slept, asking classmates and teacher if it wasn't the stereotypes that were repulsive. The closeted teacher was at a loss, and she nimbly returned classroom attention to the form of the novel, yet she felt the students had been aware of her dodge. She did not fit the stereotypes — neither did most of the students and faculty coming out — but she was afraid of how she might be judged.

Coming out felt impossible. My closeted colleague worried about her privacy: If she came out, would students speculate about her Saturday trips into town? Would she ever dare bring a "friend" back to the dorm? Worst of all, what if some female student in the locker room or the dormitory accused her of "looking" at her or "coming on" to her? Every time she saw a gay or lesbian colleague with whom she might talk about the issues, she found herself shying away. By the end of the term, she was packing her bags, unready to remain and face her personal issues.

Not everyone is ready to emerge gleefully from the closet, ready to change the world. Sometimes the inner landscape contains too many obstacles for a teacher, or a student, to face coming out with aplomb.

Many students choose, as did my colleague, to keep their secrets under wraps while still in high school. When the Homo-Bi-Heterosexual Alliance on campus hosts its yearly reunion for Northfield Mt. Hermon alumni, stories of secrecy tumble out, filling the conference room with a gusty air of relief. One of the most dramatic comings-out by an alumnus of NMH occurred just this year, when a young man called from his college dormitory to tell me all about his new-found sexuality. Actually, he confessed, he'd known as early as March of his senior year. Around campus, he had the reputation of a homophobe, despite friendships with people who later came out as bisexual. His marine crewcut and aggressive Young Republican stance against the liberal side in political arguments made him seem easy to categorize, so my face lit up with astonished delight as he told me his story. He had called to come out, because it was National Coming Out week. But he also wanted to volunteer to make a presentation at an HBH meeting sometime during the term.

I eagerly accepted his offer, then sought and received his permission to use his name on posters advertising a discussion on coming out. (Unfortunately, because of fears about parental angst, he prefers not to have his name appear in this essay.) In the capsule version of his coming out story, he mentioned that it was his reactions to stories read in his English class that made him first think about his nascent sexuality. When feelings surfaced within him that he could not explain away, when his attractions began to veer strongly toward those of his own sex, this student realized that in his homophobia he was reacting against himself.

The deeply personal nature of sexuality causes many teachers to feel doubt about the appropriateness of addressing such matters in their classes. Yet how can we isolate such a vital issue as sexuality from the intellectual sphere, from the school as a place where so many vital discoveries are made? Education needs to be about dangerous questions. Yet we teachers too often yield to our vulnerabilities and sacrifice the opportunity for English classrooms to become the crossroads where intellectual learning and the more personal complexities intersect.

The most pointed question I have ever received on the nature of what is appropriate came from an articulate, thoughtful woman who was a teacher and English curriculum supervisor in her school district. During a morning break punctuating a day full of lectures and discussions about diversity in the curriculum, she asked: Why is it necessary to include this kind of thing in an English class? As a black woman, she was sensitive to the need for various voices to be heard, yet she felt homophobic reservations. "I'm a mother and a grandmother," she said, making the issue personal right away. "I wouldn't want my grandson to learn about gay subtexts in his grade 9 English class. He might start wondering about the lifestyle, might start wondering about his own sexuality, because children at that age always want to try things. None of my family wants him trying that, I can promise you."

The only way to answer her was to address this possibility, so I did: "If your grandson is thinking he's gay, he'll find out pretty soon whether he is or not, without any help from an English class. If he's not gay, no amount of reading about gay lives will make him gay. If he is gay, no amount of silence will make him change." I went on to tell stories about the exclusion experienced by gay students who found no mention of their feelings or their dilemmas in any classroom. The veteran teacher who also was a grandmother listened closely, agreeing at last that the avoidance of prickly issues in the English classroom helps no student — gay or straight.

Personal exchanges like this one are the best way around the red herring of appropriateness. But until more teachers are able to confront one another with honest questions, vital issues will be left out of curricular planning and classroom interaction. Teachers will continue to fear the label of "inappropriate subject matter," to dodge around the definition of "what's developmentally appropriate," and never to face the complex fact that student development occurs haphazardly, that students are individuals, and that hushing certain discussions merely leaves important questions, fears, doubts, or troubles to fester in silence.

To avoid this silence, we gay and lesbian educators must bear the brunt of such questioning. But we are not completely alone. I know of at least one heterosexual teacher who, because she has a homosexual relative or friend, makes special efforts to include issues about homosexuality in class discussions. She suggested the use of the novel *Jack* by A.M. Homes as a good one for opening discussion. In this book Jack is a straight adolescent who is unhappy with his father's newfound gay identity, and the book explores the improvements in his awareness as he becomes more familiar with his father's interior and exterior life.

Interestingly, another heterosexual English teacher, whom I met at a conference, spoke of her difficulty in using *Jack* in class. Her gay brother had been struggling with coming out to his family, and certain scenes in the novel left her on the brink of tears. She felt unable to teach the book effectively because of her vulnerable feelings and deep personal associations with the subject.

However, this is precisely the sort of personal engagement that, once teachers come to terms with their own conflicts and issues, can provide the most fertile ground from which to present a lesson. While we teachers do not need to bare our souls at every juncture in the classroom, we may find that teaching from the vantage of personal knowledge will allow students to find their own difficult connections between text and life.

Perhaps it is no easier for heterosexuals to present and explore these texts and subtexts than it is for a closeted gay teacher or even for an "out" lesbian for whom the issues are personal. Difficult issues of life, often grounded exclusively in the heterosexual viewpoint, come up in discussion all the time. Love, sex, and family dynamics tend to be literary subject matter, worthy of taking a thesis on, writing a story about, or discussing in class. Why not banish fear and broaden the spectrum? Students — gay and straight — will benefit from inclusiveness of all kinds. Through inclusive teaching, we can foster self-acceptance, acceptance of others, and a literary intelligence cognizant of the many texts lurking in humankind.

Resources

Blackwomon, Julie, and Caspers, Nona. *Voyages Out 2: Lesbian Short Fiction*. Seattle: Seal Press, 1990.

Homes, A.M. *Jack*. New York: Macmillan, 1989.

Koppelman, Susan, ed. *Between Mothers and Daughters*. New York: Feminist Press of CUNY, 1985.

Leavitt, David. *Family Dancing*. New York: Alfred A. Knopf, 1984.

Mishima, Yukio *Confessions of a Mask*. Translated by Meredith Weatherby. New York: New Directions, 1985.

Salinger, J.D. *The Catcher in the Rye*. New York: Little, Brown, 1951.

Walker, Alice. *The Color Purple*. New York: Harcourt Brace Jovanovich, 1982.

The Sussex Program and Its Contexts

by Alan Sinfield

MPs Slam 'Degree in Gays'

Students at a university are being offered a degree course in gay and lesbian studies. But the one year course at Sussex University in Brighton is under attack by Tory MPs. Terry Dicks said it was a waste of taxpayers' subsidy. "The place should be shut down and disinfected," he said.

(*Daily Mirror*, 25 February 1991.)

The press got hold of the Sussex English MA program, "Sexual Dissidence and Cultural Change," in February 1991, in the middle of the tabloid assault on persons with AIDS, and a couple of years after the infamous Section 28 became law, prohibiting municipalities from spending money on projects that "promote homosexuality." Nonetheless, as I write this in spring 1995, the fourth intake of the Sussex MA is halfway through.

In England, male homosexuality has been legal since 1967, provided that you are in private, there are only two of you, and you are over 18 years old (changed in 1994 from 21). Lesbianism is not illegal. Western Europe generally is similar; in some countries the age of consent is lower.

Section 28 was an attempt to rein back the growth of lesbian and gay subcultures. A sponsor of the law reform of 1967 declared: "Any form of ostentatious behavior, any form of public flaunting, would be utterly disgraceful

93

and make the sponsors of the Bill regret what they have done."[1] The current situation was unthinkable at that time — bars, cafés, and bookstores, manifestly gay and open to the street; widely distributed newspapers, books, and videos. We've been flaunting it.

Section 28 does not signal a simple state of homophobic reaction in the United Kingdom. On the one hand, it is only one part of a wider attack, under the Thatcher and Major Conservative administrations, on relatively democratic or autonomous institutions of civil society, such as municipalities, television and radio, trade unions, schools, and universities. On the other hand, it is significantly contested — as the change in the age of consent for men from 21 to 18, which passed through parliament on a free vote after a vigorous campaign, indicates. In fact, Section 28 was largely counterproductive, for it politicized a generation that had become complacent with its discos and decor; and it was the ground of an unprecedented alliance between lesbians and gay men, who were drawn together by the fact that, for the first time, they were legislated against together.

In the same period, there has been a new flourishing of lesbian and gay commerce with the development of gay business districts in cities such as London, Manchester, and Brighton.

This uneven situation may best be understood through a distinction drawn by David T. Evans, in his important book, *Sexual Citizenship*.[2] The 1967 law reform deployed a new distinction: between legality and morality. Despite the legalizing of many gay sexual practices in private, the alleged immorality of lesbians and gay men remains, seeming to justify the withholding of citizenship rights in numerous respects, especially in what might seem parts of the private sphere, such as familial and quasifamilial contexts (partnership rights, parenting, fostering, schools, entertainment in the home). In fact, lesbians and gay men may be regarded as the vanguard of the coming phase of capitalism, in which citizenship will amount to little more than an invitation to consume and pay taxes.

Section 28 does not apply to universities and probably does not apply to high schools. (The situation is unclear). However, high schools recently have been subject to government regulation designed to inhibit the discussion of lesbian and gay matters, including the dangers of the HIV virus. Homosexuality may be legal, but that does not mean that the state intends to give it any encouragement. The deficiencies in official policies on AIDS advice in the UK all boil down to one issue: The state cannot bear to *recommend* safe gay practices. Lately the government has introduced a rule whereby parents are invited to withdraw their children from sex education. Now, if parents were told, "There is a fair chance — 1 in 10, 1 in 20, it makes little difference — that your son will engage in gay sexual practices, so do you want him to learn how to avoid catching a life-threatening condition?" almost all would say, "Yes." But that is not how the question is posed. Parents are told: "Gays are other people, gays are disgusting, even your innocent child might be at risk of seduction if anyone mentions, with other than shock and horror, that there is more than one kind of sexuality."

The university system in the UK is entirely within the public sector. Its development since 1945 has been within an "arm's length" of relative autonomy, with a view to protecting the independence of research and scholarship. Under Conservative administrations since 1979, a high level of interference has occurred. Even so, the ideology of independent scholarship remains powerful, and research in humanities is relatively untrammeled. There is every reason to suppose that government ministers would not welcome any substantial development of lesbian and gay studies, but it would not appear reasonable to interfere with the present level of activity.

There are options in lesbian and gay studies (undergraduate and postgraduate) at perhaps one in five universities; Essex, Loughborough, Warwick, York, and the London colleges, Birkbeck and Queen Mary and Westfield, are prominent.[3] However, the MA at the University of Sussex is still the only entire degree course.

The question that's always asked is how we got it through, and we still don't altogether know. We just prepared the paperwork very carefully and submitted it through the system. The English subject group (approximately, the department) were enthusiastic; higher committees passed it without comment. *And why shouldn't they?* Prestigious North American schools and presses are doing it. Sussex faculty and students are notoriously progressive and innovative, and the English curriculum displays ongoing interdisciplinary, feminist, postcolonial, cultural materialist, and theoretical concerns. The proposers were tenured and promoted, were publishing in lesbian and

. . . apart from the initial tabloid hysteria, there have been very few hostile comments.

95

gay studies with reputable presses, and already had research students working on sexualities. Gay options already were being taught in the other English MA programs. We required no structural change and threatened no one's patch.

Only subsequently did we realize how lucky we must have been. Influential university administration figures must have been preoccupied; for as soon as the press picked up the story, they came out (or, rather, went in) as very edgy indeed. We found that the press office was trying to handle the matter without any reference to the relevant faculty. They evidently regarded us as an embarrassment. (Later we got onto better terms with them and they proved a big help.) When an additional option was passed by the subject group, it was held up on a sequence of pretexts, none of which could be sustained. After the then-vice chancellor resigned, we were told that he had been personally distressed about the topic.

Recent changes of personnel in the university administration and the achievement by the English subject group of the top grade in a national exercise to evaluate research achievement have produced a more positive climate. In 1994 a new post with expertise in lesbian studies was established, enabling us to round out the course offerings with a full option on lesbian theory. About a dozen postgraduates currently are writing doctoral dissertations at Sussex on themes to do with sexualities. And we run "Queory," a seminar open to all members of the university, with a circulation list of 100 and average attendance of 40.

What all this shows is that, in the UK, you can do lesbian and gay studies 1) if you get the breaks and 2) at some risk. In fact, apart from the initial tabloid hysteria, there have been very few hostile comments. There is a question, though, about how much professional development will be possible. Lesbian and gay studies are not going to be as big as feminism because they do not have the potential appeal to half the population (though perhaps they should). At first sight they might seem comparable with Black Studies, but most of our undergraduate constituency, at 18 to 21 years of age, are not used to being lesbian or gay and may be afraid to commit themselves to a special study.

The MA at most UK universities is a one-year course with two principal constituencies. For some students, it is the opportunity to "top up and round off," in a more specialized way, skills and topics that were broached in their

Not everyone is happy to see the academy moving on lesbian and gay literary culture.

96

BA degree. For others, it is a basis for subsequent doctoral research (Ph.D. study in the UK normally requires little or no coursework). The English MA at Sussex has an intake of about 80 students each year, about the same as the BA intake. It is an intensive one-year course, all in small-group teaching. MA students are a forceful and lively presence; they set a good deal of the intellectual tone of the subject group.

Between 10 and 20 students enroll annually for Sexual Dissidence, which is one of five English programs; the others are Renaissance, Critical Theory, Literary History and Cultural Discourse, and Twentieth Century. There is a lot of interaction between the programs. Some courses appear in more than one program, and students may take courses from programs other than the one for which they enroll. Students take four courses out of a choice of 10: two in the autumn, two in the spring. In the summer they write a dissertation.

The options and tutors are: Sexuality, Transgression and Subcultures (Jonathan Dollimore); Lesbianism and Literature (Sandra Freeman); Male Homosexuality and Literature (Alan Sinfield); Feminist Criticisms and Contemporary Women's Writing (Jenny Taylor); Sexuality/Sexual Difference (Mandy Merck); Theatre and Homosexual Representation (Alan Sinfield); Homosexuality, Film and TV: Representations and Readings (Andy Medhurst); Restoration and Eighteenth Century Constructions of Sexuality (Siobhan Kilfeather); The Lesbian Subject (Rachel Holmes); and Dissidence and Marginality in the Theatre of Shakespeare and His Contemporaries (Jonathan Dollimore).

Prominent publications by members of the course team include: Rachel Bowlby, *Shopping with Freud* (Routledge, 1993); Jonathan Dollimore, *Sexual Dissidence* (Oxford University Press, 1991); Mandy Merck, *Perversions: Deviant Readings* (Virago, 1993); Alan Sinfield, *The Wilde Century* (Columbia, 1994); and *Cultural Politics — Queer Reading* (University of Pennsylvania Press, 1994).

I believe almost all the students in the program have had a rewarding time. They are more committed than the average run of postgraduate students. Some have been struggling for two years to get lesbian or gay material into undergraduate courses; some are returners who have been running helplines, reading groups, and so on. They see a lot of each other, sometimes quite intensely. The university is on the edge of Brighton, an atmospheric old seaside town with a large traditional gay community.

It is not difficult to get an MA place at Sussex if you have a good first degree, not necessarily in English. But it is expensive. The university has virtually no resources with which to support students, and the government insists on high fees (though not as high as those usually charged in the USA). If you want to know more about the university and its programs, write to Postgraduate Admissions, Sussex House, University of Sussex, Brighton, BN1 9RH, England.

Let me conclude by voicing an anxiety that is perhaps particularly European. Not everyone is happy to see the academy moving on lesbian and gay literary culture. There are two, divergent reasons. One is that many gay men have found the "man of letters" tradition rewarding. Richard Dyer writes of his younger self: "Queerness brought with it artistic sensitivity, it gave you the capacity to appreciate and respond to culture. It was a compensation for having been born or made queer. . . . It also made you doubly 'different' — queer and cultured. And how splendid to be different! Even if you were awful."[4]

A second reason for anxiety about gaining academic status is that, in our desire to become academically acceptable, our politics may become submerged in professional criteria. Hazel Carby, in *Reconstructing Womanhood*, complains about this in regard to Black feminist criticism, which "for the main part accepts the prevailing paradigms predominant in the academy, as has women's studies and Afro-American studies, and seeks to organize itself as a discipline in the same way."[5] It has been depressing to watch North American lesbian and gay studies getting incorporated into the academic star system, which requires that an individual who makes a notable contribution be hugely feted and rewarded, so that in the ensuing phase everyone else can feel justified in gathering round and attacking him or her, thereby establishing their own positions.

This is perhaps easier to say from the UK, where lesbian and gay studies are unthinkable outside a general left-wing orientation, and hence are accompanied by a serious suspicion of the market, cultural hierarchy, and the education system as an ideological state apparatus or bank of cultural capital, and hence of conventional English studies. We feel uneasy at institutional success and love that Walter Benjamin quote about there being "no document of civilization which is not at the same time a document of barbarism."[6] Anyway, we don't have the money to sustain a star system.

With these factors in mind, we need to work specifically to keep lesbian and gay studies in touch with wider lesbian and gay subcultures. Therefore I propose a shift in self-conceptualization, away from the category, English literature professionals engaged in lesbian and gay studies, toward the category, lesbian and gay intellectuals.

Antonio Gramsci is a good reference point here because he acknowledges that all people are intellectual and endorses a wisdom in common sense while also specifying as a social category the people who perform the social functions of intellectuals. Gramsci distinguishes organic and traditional intellectuals. The former are organic to their class, whereas the latter, who in his society were mostly gentlemen of means, "put themselves forward as autonomous and independent of the dominant social group." One way of making political ground is to capture the traditional intellectuals, but "ideally," Gramsci says, "the proletariat should be able to generate its own 'organic' intellectuals within the class who remain intellectuals *of* their class."[7] Of course, academics can turn out for a demonstration like other people. My demand is more specific: that the lesbian and gay movements generate organic intellectuals.

Lesbian and gay people need subculture.

To be sure, as Michel Foucault observes, it has become difficult to work as an intellectual at all without becoming enmeshed in a profession.[8] I am proposing a priority: that we try to stop thinking of lesbian and gay studies as a sufficient objective. Ask not what we can do for the academy, but whether it can do anything for lesbian and gay people.

This is not to say that we should withdraw from organized study. Rather, it is because exclusivity is impossible — because the academy is so powerful and because gayness is so inextricably involved with heterosexuality — that this priority needs asserting. Nor will it be a matter just of writing different kinds of academic papers. We have to discover further institutional opportunities. I am particularly pleased with my column in *Gay Times*, every two or three months, in which I attempt to review new academic books in an accessible way.

Recently, Richard Rorty has tried to distinguish a wrong and a right kind of multiculturalism. It is admirable that black children should learn about Frederick Douglass, Harriet Tubman, and W.E.B. Du Bois, he says, but this may end up with "the dubious recommendation that a black child should be brought up in a special culture, one peculiar to blacks." Rorty does not want black children to feel that "their culture is not that of their white schoolmates, that they have no share in the mythic America imagined by the Founders and by Emerson and Whitman, the America partially realized by Lincoln and by King."[9] Up to a point this is surely right, but Rorty allows subculture to sound like an optional extra. Rather, it is an invaluable defensive strategy. A very common feature of coming-out narratives, still, is terror at being the only one, for it seems inconceivable that mainstream representations of lesbians and gay men might comprise oneself. As Stuart Hall remarks of colonial regimes, "They had the power to make us see and experience *ourselves* as 'Other'."[10]

Subculture is not just where oppression is registered and resisted, it is where self-under-standings . . . may be explored and re-made.

Lesbian and gay people need subculture. The dominant ideology sustains itself by constituting subjectivities that will find "natural" its view of the world (hence its dominance). Subcultures tend to constitute partially alternative subjectivities. In that bit of the world where the subculture rules, you may feel confident, as we used to say, that black is beautiful, gay is good. "In acquiring one's conception of the world one belongs to a particular grouping which is that of all the social elements which share the same mode of thinking and acting," Antonio Gramsci observes.[11] It is through such sharing — through interaction with others who are engaged with compatible preoccupations — that one may develop a workable alternative subject position.

Put simply, subculture is good for morale. Considered as a model for the good society, a gay disco lacks quite a lot. But for a gay man it is a place where he is in the majority, where some of his values and assumptions rule. Of course, it is a fantasy world, as he knows all too well from the street aggression as he enters and leaves. But, by so much, it is a space of sharing and reassurance. Further, subculture is where we may address, on terms that make sense to us, the problems that confront us; where we may work on our own confusions, conflicts and griefs. There are problems enough — in our relations with straight cultures and, at least as important, among ourselves — matters of misogyny, bisexuality, and sado-masochism; class, racial, and inter-generational exploitation; HIV and AIDS.

Subculture is not just where oppression is registered and resisted, it is where self-understandings — fraught, as they inevitably are, with the self-oppression that stigma produces — may be explored and re-made. The task for lesbian and gay intellectuals will not be establishing a correct line, but using our privileges of time and money and our hard-won academic skills to illuminate histories and problems.

References

1. Quoted in Tim Newburn, *Permission and Regulation* (London: Routledge, 1992), p.60.
2. David T. Evans, *Sexual Citizenship* (London: Routledge, 1993), pp. 50-54.
3. For a list of UK academics and courses, write to DOLAGS, Unit 64, Eurolink Centre, 49 Effra Rd., London, SW2 1BZ.
4. Derek Cohen and Richard Dyer, "The Politics of Gay Culture," in *Power and Politics*, edited by the Gay Left Collective (London: Allison and Busby, 1980), p. 177.
5. Hazel V. Carby, *Reconstructing Womanhood* (New York: Oxford University Press, 1987), pp. 15-16.
6. Walter Benjamin, *Illuminations* (Glasgow: Collins, 1973), p. 258.
7. Antonio Gramsci, *Selections from the Prison Notebooks*, translated by Quintin Hoare and Geoffrey Nowell Smith (London: Lawrence and Wishart, 1971), pp. 6-7, 10.
8. Michel Foucault, *Power/Knowledge*, edited by Colin Gordon (Brighton; Harvester, 1980), pp. 126-33. I discuss these issues further in *Cultural Politics — Queer Reading* (Philadelphia: Pennsylvania University Press, and London: Routledge, 1994).
9. Richard Rorty, "A Leg-Up for Oliver North," *London Review of Books*, 20 October 1994, pp. 13, 15.
10. Stuart Hall, "Cultural Identity and Diaspora," in *Identity: Community, Culture, Difference*, edited by Jonathan Rutherford (London: Lawrence and Wishart, 1990), p. 225.
11. Gramsci, *Selections from the Prison Notebooks*, p. 324.

Agency and Identity in the Gay and Lesbian Studies Classroom: A Perspective from Australia

by David Phillips*

In an interview first published in 1981 Michel Foucault poses the question, "Is it possible to create a homosexual mode of life?" He adds, "To be 'gay,' I think, is not to identify with the psychological traits and the visible masks of the homosexual, but to try to define and develop a way of life."[1] Remarks such as these might be viewed as indicative of "the liquidation of the principle of identity" that often has been cited as a central concern in Foucault's writings.[2]

However, Foucault's skepticism regarding identity, and identity politics generally, should be placed in the context of the emphasis in his later work on the individual's self-creation, or *ascesis*, an emphasis that can be viewed in part as a redress against the social constructionist position with which Foucault is more readily identified. Thus, for example, as Foucault explains at the beginning of the interview:

*The author wishes to thank his colleagues, Frances Bonner and Bronwen Levy, for their comments and contributions to an earlier version of this paper, published as "Pedagogy, Theory, and the Scene of Resistance" in *Radical Teacher* 45 (Winter 1994): 38-41. The author also thanks Clive Kanes, Patrick Palmer, and Michael Metcalfe.

Another thing to distrust is the tendency to relate the question of homosexuality to the problem of "Who am I?" and "What is the secret of my desire?" Perhaps it would be better to ask oneself, "What relations, through homosexuality, can be established, invented, multiplied and modulated?" The problem is not to discover in oneself the truth of sex but rather to use sexuality henceforth to arrive at a multiplicity of relationships. And no doubt that's the real reason why homosexuality is not a form of desire but something desirable.[3] Therefore we have to work at becoming homosexuals and not be obstinate in recognizing that we are.

This stress on homosexuality as something to be created or invented is reiterated by Foucault in another interview given three years later, in which he states:

Sexuality is something that we ourselves create — it is our own creation, and much more than the discovery of a secret side of our desire. We have to understand that with our desires, through our desires, go new forms of relationships, new forms of love, new forms of creation. Sex is not a fatality; it's a possibility for creative life. . . . We don't have to discover that we are homosexuals. . . . Rather, we have to create a gay life. To *become*.[4]

One year after Foucault's 1981 interview, Eric Michaels, an American anthropologist working in Australia, also questioned the consequences of adopting an identity — not so much rejecting identity, as such, but rather resisting contemporary (commodified) forms of gay identity. Michaels noted that:

What bothers me is that being a faggot isn't very interesting any more. When I walk into a disco, or a bar, or a baths, I don't feel I'm entering any kind of new age. I don't feel I'm on the frontier. We're not avant-garde any more. We're not avant anything. We imitate everybody else now. They don't imitate us. . . . I liked being deviant.[5]

Here Michaels is rejecting what he sees as the normalizing effects of the commercial expansion of gay culture and the concomitant emergence of a gay ghetto. These, he argues, have led to an absence of social criticism, "for that's what the gay sensibility was; a critical perspective on American life and values." To counter this domesticated assimilation of gay life, Michaels calls for a project of historical reclamation: "We need to take some responsibility for our own history, for conveying it to our young. It's not nostalgia. If one is going to go to all the trouble of being gay, one ought to do a more interesting and useful job of it. Models exist in our very recent past. They should be recalled."[6]

While we may not necessarily agree with the commentary that Michaels presents, what is at issue in both his and Foucault's observations is the heuristic value of identity. More specifically, though commenting from different perspectives, both are rejecting reified forms of identity. These, they claim, have become obstacles to an exploration of homosexuality's transformative potential. In short, for both Foucault and Michaels, the significance of homosexuality lies principally in its capacity for reconfiguring existing social relations and for generating new ones. Thus, just as Michaels bemoans the reduction of a gay liberationist agenda to an almost exclusive concern with consumption (sexual or otherwise), so too, for Foucault, the impact of homosexuality lies in its "formation of new alliances and the tying together of unforeseen lines of force. . . that's what makes homosexuality 'disturbing': the homosexual mode of life much more than the sexual act itself."[7]

Taking my cue from the comments of Foucault and Michaels, my concern here is to address some of the pedagogic implications arising from these descriptions of homosexuality as a potentiality and process rather than an identity, as "becoming gay" rather than "being gay." More specifically, I wish to posit a distinction between agency (becoming) and identity (being) in relation to social constructionism, which is now the dominant paradigm, indeed orthodoxy, within gay and lesbian cultural studies.

Despite the enormous appeal of social constructionism, its dominance is very much contained within academe. Indeed, even within the university, its claims often are met with perplexity and, at times, hostility from students. My concern is to address what this resistance might tell us of the limitations of social constructionism both within the classroom and within society more generally. In part because of its own omissions, social constructionism may in fact have some disabling effects, both pedagogically and politically. Moreover, if much current gay and lesbian theory is alienating many of its intended constituents, this alienation undermines the very rationale of gay

. . . social construc- tionism may in fact have some disabling effects . . .

and lesbian studies. In short, what do we (as both teachers and students) see as the purpose of gay and lesbian studies?

A recognition of the disabling effects of social constructionism is implicit in the now commonplace observation that contemporary gay and lesbian cultural studies and theory are premised on an apparent contradiction. While critiquing the essentialism behind various versions of identity politics, gay and lesbian cultural studies must simultaneously retrieve or preserve some notion of identity. This tension between the political and pedagogic need for identity and the contingency of sexual identities raises significant questions for the teaching of gay and lesbian studies. My concern here is with the effects of this contradiction on classroom practice in terms of the problems that may arise when teaching a course that seeks to affirm lesbian and gay identities but that also employs theory that challenges dominant or "commonsense" accounts of identity.

"Teaching, like analysis," argues Shoshana Felman, "has to deal not so much with lack of knowledge as with resistances to knowledge. Ignorance . . . is a passion . . . [and] is nothing other than a desire to ignore; its nature is less cognitive than performative."[8] If, as Felman implies, teaching is enacted within a scene of resistance involving "an active dynamic of negation, an active refusal of information," my specific focus is on the forms of resistance that may be encountered in the classroom to the theoretical critiques of identity offered by social constructionism. I shall address this resistance to theory on two levels. First, to what extent is it a function of the theory itself? For example, is theory perceived as a threat to the presumed integrity of subjectivity and identity whereby resistance involves, as Felman describes it, "the incapacity — or the refusal — to acknowledge one's own implication in the information"? But here I also wish to think about what the resistance to theory might indicate about the limitations of social constructionism itself, both within the teaching of gay and lesbian studies and as a platform to oppose homophobic accounts of sexual identity formation (for example, the current scientific search for a physiological basis for homosexuality).

Second, and perhaps more important in the present context, to what extent might this resistance be a function of the pedagogic representation or performance of that theory within the classroom itself? Is resistance an issue relating more to process or method, rather than to content (the actual claims of theory)? Furthermore, might not method and content effectively contradict or negate each other?

My comments on pedagogic practice are based on observations arising from the teaching of a lesbian and gay studies course offered for the first time at the University of Queensland in 1993 and again in 1995. This undergraduate course, "Gay and Lesbian Cultures," is to my knowledge the first gay and lesbian studies course to be offered at an Australian university, though several courses currently are being planned and one or two specifically lesbian studies courses also now exist. The actual course title was a topic of some discussion among those teaching it. Some felt that an explicitly gay and lesbian title could discourage students who might be anxious about parents or friends finding out or who would not want the course title to be printed on their final grade card. But our consensus was that, if such a course was to go ahead, then the words "gay" and "lesbian" should be used instead of more oblique wording.

The existence of such a course in Australia reflects the emergence of gay and lesbian studies as an important area of recent academic innovation and publishing primarily, of course, in the United States but increasingly also in Australia. As in the United States, the emergence of gay and lesbian studies is the result largely of three factors: 1) the emergence of a visible and articulate gay culture, 2) the impact of feminism, and most recently 3) the currency (albeit still very limited) of poststructuralist theory within university humanities departments. Gay and lesbian issues also have received much political and media attention. Examples include the campaign to decriminalize male homosexuality in Tasmania, the debate over gays in the military, and the growing national and international significance of the lesbian and gay cultural events. In addition, the question of identity currently has a very high profile in Australia because of debates around issues such as republicanism, Aboriginal rights, multiculturalism, and Australia's role in the Asia-Pacific region. Indeed, the politically driven search for a distinctly Australian identity threatens to become the sole agenda in contemporary Australian culture.

Perhaps most surprising is that a gay and lesbian course should be taught first in Queensland, which has a reputation in Australia for being a politically and socially conservative — indeed, "redneck" — state. However, this conservatism also has fueled a tradition of oppositional politics and, within

Queensland's universities, a number of innovative and politicized courses (for example, around race history and women's studies). While reactionary politics certainly were the norm under the 30-year domination of Queensland by the National Party (which was unabashedly homophobic in its attitudes and policies), there has been some undoubted progress since the victory of the Labor Party in December 1989. Managerial, rather than social, reform is the major agenda of the Labor Party; and its social attitudes (on abortion, pornography, and the legalization of prostitution) still are strongly conservative by national standards. However, homosexuality has been decriminalized. This legal reform, together with equal opportunities legislation, has been fundamental in generating a climate in which a gay and lesbian studies course could even be offered at the University of Queensland. Yet the heritage of decades of right-wing state government remains. Social conservatism, indeed conformism, continues to be strong in Queensland. Arguably, this conformism is evident also in the attitudes of many gays and lesbians.

The "Gay and Lesbian Cultures" course is an interdisciplinary subject initially taught by four lecturers (two female, two male) from two departments, with myself (as convenor) from Art History and my three colleagues (one of whom is now at another university) from English. Enrollment in the course (after some students dropped out) in 1993 was 59 and is 39 in 1995, which is relatively high for an interdisciplinary course offered to students in their second year and above. The number is particularly high for the first offering of a course. About 80% of students are women, many of them already enrolled for a major in women's studies. For these students the course is an additional, optional subject. This also may account for the surprisingly high number of heterosexual students (not all of them women) in the class. Given the course prerequisites, most students would have some cultural studies background. Indeed, the majority are based in the English Department, which offers courses on literature, drama, film and television, and cultural studies. Both English and Art History also offer a range of theory, or theory-informed, courses. Exceptions to prerequisites are made for students from other disciplines, such as social work and psychology.

The majority of students also have come to university directly after completing their school education, but the course does have a broader age range than most university courses. The ethnic profile of the class is almost exclusively Caucasian and, as such, reflects the ethnic and social background of

Many students also have gone through considerable efforts to establish and articulate their sexual identities.

the vast majority of arts students. Aboriginal and Torres Strait Islander students remain a very small presence on campus across all departments, while most overseas Asian students are enrolled in more "vocational" departments, such as engineering and the various sciences.

In keeping with its title, the course focuses on gay and lesbian culture, especially the representation of homosexual identities. This is not to claim that questions of identity politics either are or should be the starting point for gay and lesbian studies or, indeed, for this particular course. But this emphasis follows in part from the training and interests of the lecturers, as we are neither social scientists, sociologists, nor historians. The course is not a history of the gay movement, nor does it explicitly address sociological and anthropological accounts of homosexuality or empirical case-studies and surveys, ethnographic approaches that have, until fairly recently, dominated academic discussions of homosexuality. While such approaches were sometimes alluded to in class by way of cultural theory, both the concern of this course and the backgrounds of those teaching it are indicative of the conjunction of lesbian and gay studies with cultural studies and theory that has marked the academic emergence of gay studies over the past few years. This conjunction, while still falling under the broad label of social constructionism, has given greater attention to the discursive production of sexuality and thus marks a shift from the concerns of earlier constructionist theory.

Taking the representation of homosexual identities as its central focus, the course is structured both thematically (for example, resistance, appropriation, coming out, the avant-garde, institutional spaces) and by topics that are of particular interest to those teaching it (such as film, drama, lesbian writing, photography). The structure of the class, which is scheduled for three hours, is a 60- to 90-minute lecture (usually by one or two lecturers) followed by tutorial discussions. By the end of the 1993 course, the tutorial groups had in fact become one large group of about 35 students — no doubt partly as a consequence of the student responses addressed here.

The Omissions of Social Constructionism

While we may be able to talk about same-sex desire or behavior existing in the past, we need to recognize how the meanings of this behavior were, and continue to be, mediated by culturally specific representations.

For constructionism, sexuality is a contextually and relationally produced effect. Thus, taking up the claims of Foucault, it could be argued that we can not even talk of sexuality as a natural phenomenon in terms, for example, of distinct desires, pleasures, and drives that are then molded by culture. Sexuality is not some innate register or subjective core, a "truth" of our being. It is produced entirely by the regulatory orderings of the society. If so, the political imperative should not be to reify historically arbitrary and fictive constructs of homosexual identity but instead to resist the classificatory identities generated by modernity. Claims for a homosexual ontology (that there is some "essential" or intrinsic homosexual identity and continuity across cultures) are thus displaced by an emphasis on the fundamentally modern emergence of the classificatory systems and categories that describe and structure sexuality. We might think instead of sexualities as a set of attributes or meanings that are adopted, acted out, performed — and resisted. As entirely a cultural, rather than an innate or natural, formation, identity is not given, innate, or fixed but is strategic, tactical and, of course, political.

Although it has had an important role in the pluralization of various homosexualities, "the virtue of social constructionism may also be its vice," as Carole Vance has suggested.[9] Despite referring to the status of the body within social constructionism, Vance's comment applies equally to the question of causality in that, while constructionism is able to delineate variable cultural and historical productions of identities, it offers no account as to why particular identities are adopted or why some individuals are homosexual. As Steven Epstein has argued, "constructionism is unable to theorize the issue of determination. . . strict constructionism implies a lack of determination in the sexual histories of individuals . . . [and] it is precisely this perceived nonvoluntary component of identity that cannot be accounted for within a strict constructionist perspective."[10]

While I do not want to argue that constructionist accounts should provide causal narratives (even if they could), the absence of such narratives induces resistance among some students. Such resistance is indicative of a more general situation in which constructionist accounts of sexual identity formation will always lose out to those accounts (for example, of a gay gene or brain, seduction theories, etc.) that claim to point to a single cause or origin for behavior. This desire for origins is a pervasive imperative in our culture and is

110

regularly encountered both within the gay and lesbian studies classroom and in public discourse more generally.[11] For this reason, any reductive or neatly causal "explanation" of sexual identity is likely to be much more readily received than a more speculative or "deconstructive" approach.

Moreover, despite its focus on the historicity of identity, social constructionism in fact provides a very static model of identity formation in that identity becomes merely the tautological and functional effect of a discursive paradigm. Such an account implicitly assumes that identity, and even sexuality, are synonymous with discourse. Yet, as Samuel Delany has argued, discourses, texts, and narratives are extremely limited sources in that "what is accepted into language at any level is *always* a highly coded, heavily policed affair. . . . The sexual experience is *still* largely outside language — at least as it (language) is constituted at any number of levels."[12] If one accepts this claim, any understanding of homosexuality almost entirely predicated on a reading of a narrow selection of literary texts will necessarily be extremely curtailed — a conclusion that also has implications for any study of gay and lesbian culture largely premised on the reading of texts and images.

Delaney's observation is echoed in part by Leo Bersani's account of how recent "gay critiques of homosexual identity have generally been *desexualizing* discourses."[13] Arguing that these critiques have initiated a "de-gaying" of gayness, Bersani asserts that "gay men and lesbians have nearly disappeared into their sophisticated awareness of how they have been *constructed as* gay men and lesbians. The discrediting of specific gay identity . . . has had the curious but predictable result of eliminating the indispensable grounds for resistance to, precisely, hegemonic regimes of the normal. We have erased ourselves in the process of denaturalizing the epistemic and political regimes that have constructed us."[14] Bersani further notes, "An assault on *any* coherent identity . . . forecloses the possibility of gay or lesbian specificity (erasing along the way the very discipline — gay and lesbian studies — within which the assault is made)."[15]

Moreover, "the agent of resistance has been erased: there is no longer any homosexual subject to oppose the homophobic subject."[16] What is especially useful here in addressing the omissions of constructionism, but without reverting to essentialism, is Bersani's claim that the positing of a gay and lesbian "specificity" (predicated on same-sex desires and practices) need not entail a "return to immobilizing definitions of identity . . . [or] to the notion of a homosexual essence. Indeed, we may discover that this particularity, in its indeterminateness and mobility, is not at all compatible with essentializing definitions."[17] In short, while specificity is retained (in part as a necessary premise for identity), this does not of itself commit us to either a privileging or reification of particular identities.

The Resistance to Theory

Paradoxically, there is within social constructionism both a recurrent focus on identity yet simultaneously too little focus. While constructionism reifies identity (as effect), it also displaces both identity (as origin) and agency (as resistance and transformation). Given this, it is not difficult to locate reasons for the hostility, or at least skepticism, to constructionism in the classroom. Many students also have gone through considerable efforts to establish and articulate their sexual identities. As a result they may find social constructionist claims to be deeply antithetical to their own beliefs. As Jeffrey Escoffier has pointed out, "Most of us start out as essentialists — that is, when we first come out, we believe that Socrates and Sappho were 'homosexuals' in the same way that lesbians or gay men of the late 20th century are homosexuals."[18] Similarly, Vance argues that, "We have all been brought up to think about sexuality in essentialist ways. . . . for all of us, essentialism was our first way of thinking about sexuality and still remains the hegemonic one in the culture."[19]

These statements point to two important issues: first, the desire for identification in the formation of sexual identity (for example, the search for others "like me" whether in the past or more currently) and, second, the continuing sway of models of origin and causality within narratives of identity formation. Social constructionism is extremely weak on both counts. Yet they are central concerns in the classroom. Not only is there a frequent tension between some students' self-perception and the implications of gay and lesbian studies, but social constructionism remains limited in terms of its ability to fulfill a desire for causal narratives and origins. As a consequence, there often is an inherent conflict between the desire of students for narratives, images, and figures of gay or lesbian identity and constructionism's denial of innate homosexual identities.

Curiously, however, the desire for mimetic identification also can operate in another direction as some students resist a historical perspective on gay and lesbian cultures by arguing that older representational strategies have nothing to do with their own contemporary experience. The demand for images and identities that are immediately "like us" thus precludes any historical overview and indeed closes off precisely the kind of perspective that Eric Michaels claimed would counter what he saw as the depoliticization of gay culture. However, this closure itself may be indicative of the possible limitations of gay and lesbian studies courses that privilege cultural theory and questions of representation and identity.

Finally, as stated, social constructionism is unable to explain why some individuals are gay or lesbian. While this demand may not be voiced quite so directly by students, the belief in an innate homosexuality underwrites the claim made by some that there is an original, or at least more "authentic," homosexual identity — for example, in claims that they already "knew" when very young that they were gay or lesbian or that they were somehow "different." Constructionism would seem to deny that conviction. However, such beliefs might be seen as compensatory ones in that their very assertion highlights the relative historical recency and social precariousness of gay and lesbian identities. As Michaels observed,

> I have always rejected the idea that gay promiscuity arises from some inherent biological drive of the male. . . . Instead, promiscuity acknowledges the fragility of gay identity, the constant necessity to reassert homosexuality precisely because it is not a persona, a practice, a sociability learned and acquired in infancy (as heterosexual forms are thought to be), rewarded and reinforced in familial and all other institutional contexts throughout childhood and youth. Homosexual forms — transactable gay identities, negotiable desires, how to be gay — probably are learned no earlier than adolescence, and often much later. . . . Gayness remains emergent in social action, and may never quite become internalized, so that each night we seek to rediscover that identity.[20]

This desire to establish an identity, and its reifying consequences, is evident in the recent adoption of "queer" as an identity label. The effects of homogenization and foreclosure that (at least in Australia) all too frequently

. . . the psychical remains largely unrecognized within social constructionism, and its absence is constructionism's greatest limitation.

113

accompany the deployment of "queer" as a tactic of naming now have partly blocked the transformative *dis*-articulation of identities that "queer" claims to initiate.[21] Nor is this foreclosure lessened by particularizing the terms of self-description through reference to gender, class, or ethnic subdivisions. Indeed, to what extent might this self-taxonomy replicate the voluntarist assumption that we are contiguous with our consciously adopted identities? Arguably, it is the asymmetries and contradictions between the various registers of subjectivity, identification, and identity that need to be addressed. These asymmetries, which cannot be fixed or subsumed by the identity labels, are disavowed when sexuality is elided with a named identity.

Thus the constant slippages in the use of "queer" often are a function not so much of a self-conscious mobility of terminology, but rather of the contradictory connotations that have attached themselves to the word. These connotations themselves are indicative of two distinct models of identity. Put schematically, there frequently is tension between an "ethnic" model of queer identity, a kind of queer essentialism, and what might be called a "deconstructive" deployment of queer that stresses the fragmentary nature of identities. From the position of this latter critique, the label "Queer Nation" itself is a potential oxymoron as it conflates an ethnic model of origins and difference with a body of theoretical work that seeks to dismantle potentially reductive models of identity.

This definitional tension is more than just a question of hermeneutics, as its effects are evident in the ways in which the citing of "queer" all too frequently collapses back into reductive accounts of identity formation on which a "deconstructive" project applies pressure. Indeed, one might argue that a hermeneutics of "queer" — the attempt to pin down and define its meanings, an attempt which parallels the taxonomic imperatives of so much identity politics, together with the adoption of "queer" as an identity label — is antithetical to those aspects of the term that are most useful strategically. Instead of pursuing an endless definition of "queer," we need to emphasize what has been called its "performative" status.[22] And, rather than conceiving of "queer" as a meaning that we can attach to persons, we might think of it as a tactical strategy and as an effect. What is strategically valuable, then, in "queer" is its generalized resistance to all claims to normativity, as well as its foregrounding of identity as difference rather than as essence.

Experience and Authority

Such reversions in the use of "queer" complement the resistance encountered in the classroom to theoretical critiques of identity in that both instances entail an attempt to fix identity by reifying categories that not only are mobile but also are means to effect change. Strategic or tactical approaches to identity are thus displaced by essentialist and teleological models. As a result, the enabling potential of identity categories becomes an obstacle to critique and transformation.

However, this issue and the validity of these responses aside, my focus is as much on the teaching of theory as a possible reason for resistance to it. This resistance can be discussed usefully in relation to two terms — experience and authority. Both terms relate to the ways in which students in the "Gay and Lesbian Cultures" course engaged with theoretical texts. For example, aside from the sheer density of many of the texts that discouraged some students from the outset, many students found the texts to be overly abstract or even mystifying. This response also echoed a recurrent claim that theory is irrelevant to the demands of political activism or "real life." Others, however, were rather dismissive of politics, which they identified with an old-fashioned reformist agenda and overly bureaucratic structures.

Textual density aside, the tone of critique in many texts led some students to read them as being overtly proscriptive, even censorial. Several students commented that they thought "experience" was now a forbidden word and that their own experiences and observations would have no place in class or, at best, would have only a subordinate status in relation to theory.[23] Thus the potentially most valuable resource in the classroom — students' own experiences — was perceived by some as being marginalized or redundant. However, many students, especially third-year and fourth-year honors students, readily took to theory, while others may have seen "abstract" theory precisely as a way to avoid having to talk about their own experiences.

But this said, an emphasis on experience actively silenced some students. As Diane Fuss has pointed out, "Experience . . . while providing some students with a platform from which to speak can also relegate other students to the sideline. Exclusion of this sort often breeds exclusivity."[24] Certainly, the dropout rate from tutorials was partly a consequence of many students

115

feeling awkward in the presence of their more articulate peers — those who, as Fuss describes them, are "in the know." (Most of these students already knew each other socially from the gay and lesbian student group on campus.) Non-attendance also resulted from students increasingly over-committing themselves with excessive course enrollments and work loads in order to complete their degrees as swiftly and economically as possible. Several students also commented privately that they simply did not have the personal knowledge (and with it the confidence) to speak about gay culture and politics. This was the situation for many of the heterosexual students who were unable to call on specifically gay or lesbian experiences or cultural forms.

> *. . . theory should not prohibit experience, but should enable its fuller articulation.*

However, many of the gay and lesbian students themselves seemed surprisingly unfamiliar with aspects of contemporary gay and lesbian culture, such as current cinema, which made calling on experience a frustrating exercise. Focusing on texts in the tutorials, rather than the experience and consumption of culture and lifestyles, provided a possible tactic to relieve this silencing of those students who, to use Fuss' description, "perceived [themselves] to be outside the magic circle."

Using experience as a classroom resource also raised other problems. Fuss argues, "The appeal to experience as the ultimate test of all knowledge, merely subtends the fantasy of autonomy and control. Belief in the truth of Experience is as much an ideological production as a belief in the authority of Truth."[25] At issue here was a conflict between a perceived agenda of the course and the students' self-perception and desire for identity or affirmation. This conflict may have been especially acute for younger students trying to put together some kind of identity or set of references for themselves. For these students, a critique of identity was not particularly welcome.

Yet, while critiques of the "authority of experience" were addressed in the course, the very process of teaching (in particular, the lecture format) effectively reinstalled a notion of authority by enforcing notions of "mastery" and "expertise," the apparent promotion of "correct" theoretical positions, as well as the authority and legitimizing status of theory itself. Thus, while much of the content of lectures emphasized unfixity, contingency, and undecidability, the rhetoric and mode of presentation could appear reductive, inflexible, and full of certainties. To an extent, this reductivism was a consequence of the need to explicate and paraphrase the arguments of complex texts; but the reiteration of essential points may well have produced an effect of dogmatism even if the opposite was intended.

This effect of reductivism also may have arisen because a critique of identity can make sense only if students have some grasp of what is actually meant by identity. Discussing particular representations from the very start of the course might have allowed more general theoretical questions to arise from them while also enabling the coincidences and connections between theory and experience to become apparent. For example, overtly declaratory or self-conscious texts, images, or even dress codes could be cited as instances of constructed or performed identities. This is not to employ cultural production as a demonstration of theory. Rather, it is to argue that the claims of theory are in many ways descriptive. Working from texts and images to theory could possibly have minimized the implication that somehow one has to "get the theory right" before looking at cultural products.

This perception that the "correct" theory had to be established before the course could continue led some students to become more preoccupied with trying to grasp what were seen as the distinct theoretical positions of the lecturers (which in fact were fairly congruent) than with addressing the broader arguments. However, other students felt that the participation of several lecturers in each class session helped undermine the idea that there was or could be a single theoretical position. While theoretical pluralism should, of course, be promoted, another objective of teaching could be to stage theory so as to avoid presenting it, even if inadvertently, as an apparently seamless body of knowledge. Staging contradictions, both between theory and experience and within experience, could then draw on the observations, identifications, and desires of participants in the class but without naturalizing or reifying them. One example of this strategy might be a focus on various forms of political activism, especially AIDS activism and related cultural production, which, as several students noted, could have had greater prominence in the course. Here, as in the "queer" debate, questions of subjectivity and identity, agency and representation, and the redefinition of the political are not abstract issues but are unavoidable considerations with the concerns of theory being intrinsic to representation just as experience and identity are themselves always theory-laden.

If both the articulation and the silencing of experience within the classroom present no easy resolution, the situation is potentially even more difficult when seeking to directly engage with identification and desire. Yet some engagement with the psychical is fundamental both to the agenda and pedagogy of lesbian and gay cultural studies.[26] The psychical remains largely unrecognized within social constructionism, and its absence is constructionism's greatest limitation. Indeed, a focus on the psychical (and with it questions of agency and the specificity of experience) could prevent social constructionism from lapsing into crude functionalist models that close off its political efficacy. The business of gay and lesbian theory is not so much a project of destabilizing identity by showing how it is constructed, but rather it is one of demonstrating that sexuality and identity themselves are destabilizing.

If the assertion of sexuality must simultaneously be the ruination of identity, this collapse (and its "theoretical" representation) might serve as a precondition for the emergence of other identities and modes of experience, thereby enabling what Teresa de Lauretis has described as "the imaging and enacting of new forms of community."[27] From this perspective we might think of homosexuality not solely as an identity or as a naming, but as a horizon of possibilities — as a potentiality and a "becoming" — that can serve to critique the present by signaling the possibility of other sexual and social relations and of other spaces for their enacting — spaces and relations that, as yet, we can scarcely imagine, let alone describe. Such a project of potentiation must exist uneasily with any notion of identity, not least because we necessarily cannot know in advance what these unrealized social arrangements might entail. However, within this creation of gay and lesbian lives, theory should not prohibit experience, but should enable its fuller articulation.

References

1. Michel Foucault, "Friendship as a Way of Life," translated by John Johnston, in *Foucault Live*, edited by Sylvère Lotringer (New York, Semiotexte, 1989), p. 207. The original interview, "De L'Amitié comme mode de vie," was published in *Le Gai Pied* 25 (April 1981), pp. 38-39.
2. Pierre Klossowki, "Digression à partir d'un portrait apocryphe," quoted in David Macey, *The Lives of Michel Foucault* (London, Hutchinson, 1993), p. xv.
3. Foucault, "Friendship as a Way of Life," op. cit., pp. 203-204. The last sentence in French reads, "Nous avons donc a nous acharner à devenir homosexuels et non pas à nous ob-

stiner a reconnaitre que nous le sommes," "De L'Amitie comme mode de vie," op. cit., p. 38.

4. "Sex, Power, and the Politics of Identity," *The Advocate* 400 (August 1984): 27, emphasis in original. Foucault also states in this interview that, "if identity becomes *the* problem of sexual existence, and if people think that they have to 'uncover' their 'own identity,' and that their own identity has to become the law, the principle, the code of their existence; if the perennial question they ask is 'Does this thing conform to my identity?' then, I think, they will turn back to a kind of ethics very close to the old heterosexual virility. If we are asked to relate to the question of identity, it has to be an identity to our unique selves. But the relationships we have to have with ourselves are not ones of identity, rather they must be relationships of differentiation, of creation, of innovation. To be the same is really boring." Ibid., p. 28, emphasis in original.

5. Eric Michaels, "Endnote," in *Unbecoming: An Aids Diary* (Rose Bay, NSW: Empress, 1990), p. 191.

6. Ibid., p. 192.

7. Foucault, "Friendship as a Way of Life," op. cit., p. 205.

8. Shoshana Felman, "Psychoanalysis and Education: Teaching Terminable and Interminable," in *Jacques Lacan and the Adventure of Insight* (Cambridge, Mass.: Harvard University Press, 1987), p. 79.

9. Carole Vance, "Social Construction Theory: Problems in the History of Sexuality," in *Homosexuality, Which Homosexuality?* (London, GMP, 1989), p. 23.

10. Steven Epstein, "Gay Politics, Ethnic Identity: The Limits of Social Constructionism," *Socialist Review* 17, no. 3 (1987): 23-24. Reprinted in *Forms of Desire*, edited by Edward Stein (New York: Routledge, 1992).

11. Jacques Derrida's sustained critique of the "metaphysics of presence" would be the most obvious reference here. See, for example, his discussion of structure and origin in "Structure, Sign and Play in the Discourse of the Human Sciences," in *Writing and Difference*, translated by Alan Bass (London: Routledge, 1978).

12. Samuel Delaney, "Aversion/Perversion/Diversion," in *Negotiating Lesbian and Gay Subjects*, edited by Monica Dorenkamp and Richard Henke (New York: Routledge, 1995), p. 28, emphases in original.

13. Leo Bersani, *Homos* (Cambridge, Mass.: Harvard University Press, 1995), p. 5, emphasis in original. See especially Chap. 2, "The Gay Absence," pp. 11-76.

14. Ibid., p. 4, emphasis in original.

15. Ibid., p. 48, emphasis in original.

16. Ibid., p. 56.

17. Ibid., p. 76.

18. Jeffrey Escoffier, "Generations and Paradigms: Mainstreams in Lesbian and Gay Studies," in *Gay and Lesbian Studies*, edited by Henry L. Minton (Binghamton, New York: Harrington Park Press, 1992), p. 17.

19. Vance, op. cit., p. 14.

20. Michaels, op. cit., p. 99. *Unbecoming* is a pertinent text in this context in that while Michaels clearly espouses a social constructionist position, he repeatedly asserts his own agency in terms, for example, of his constant resistance to various forms of social positioning.

21. This containment of "queer" is symptomatic of a difference between "queer" in Australia as distinct from America; the U.S. "queer" has had emphatically political connotations and effects. Arguably, this political dimension of critique has not been maintained in Australia, where "queer" operates more as a set of increasingly commodified cultural styles. The frequent co-opting of "queer" in Australia as a stable, uniform, and largely unexamined descriptive term (that can be attached to persons) is itself indicative of the dominance of identity issues within current cultural and political debates.

22. See, for example, Eve Kosofsky Sedgwick, "Queer Performativity: Henry James's *The Art of the Novel*," *GLQ: A Journal of Lesbian and Gay Studies* 1, no. 1 (1993): 1-16; and, in the same volume, Judith Butler, "Critically Queer," pp. 17-32, (reprinted in modified form in *Bodies That Matter*, op. cit., pp. 223-42).

23. The text I particularly have in mind here is Joan Scott's "The Evidence of Experience," reprinted in *The Lesbian and Gay Studies Reader*, edited by Henry Abelove et al. (New York: Routledge, 1993), pp. 397-415, but these comments would apply to many others. Of course, my own presentation of various "observations" of classroom practice is itself susceptible to Scott's critique of visuality and knowledge.

24. Diane Fuss, *Essentially Speaking: Feminism, Nature and Difference* (New York: 1989), p. 115.

25. Ibid., p. 114.

26. Space precludes a detailed discussion here of mimesis, identification, and desire and of their place within the gay and lesbian studies classroom, but such a discussion might start with Judith Butler's analysis of mimesis and identity in *Gender Trouble* (New York: Routledge, 1990). See also Mikkel Borch-Jacobsen's *The Freudian Subject*, translated by Catherine Porter (London: MacMillan, 1989) and *The Emotional Tie: Psychoanalysis, Mimesis and Affect*, translated by Douglas Brick et al. (Stanford, Calif.: Stanford University Press, 1992), as well as Constance Penley, "Teaching in Your Sleep: Feminism and Psychoanalysis," in *The Future of an Illusion* (London: Routledge, 1989) and Ruth Leys, "The Real Miss Beauchamp: Gender and the Subject of Imitation," in *Feminists Theorize the Political*, edited by Judith Butler and Joan Scott (New York: Routledge, 1992). See also Joan Copjec, *Read My Desire* (Cambridge, Mass.: MIT Press 1994), especially "Introduction: Structures Don't March in the Streets," pp. 1-4.

27. Teresa de Lauretis, "Queer Theory: Lesbian and Gay Sexualities, An Introduction," *Differences* 2 (Summer 1991): xvi.

Setting the Record *Less* Straight: My Skirmish with the Religious Right in Montana*

by Henry Gonshak

When I proposed a summer course on gay and lesbian studies at the Montana College of Mineral Science and Technology, where I teach English, the last thing I expected was to wind up in *USA Today*. But when a fundamentalist Christian pastor in our small, blue-collar, largely conservative town of Butte tried to have the class canceled, a furor erupted that so reverberated it eventually caught the attention of the national media.

Let me admit from the outset: My story is not quite a profile in courage. In fighting to save my class, I made mistakes; my determination sometimes wavered. Still, I think my failures, as much as my successes, may prove instructive.

I'm sure my experience isn't unique in academe, and I suspect that, unfortunately, it will become more common in the future. As our culture wars continue, the religious right is likely to expand its censorious crusades from public elementary and high schools to state-run colleges and universities. And if any one subject proves most contentious, it is sure to be the burgeoning field of gay and lesbian studies.

---

*An early version of this essay appeared as a point-of-view piece, "A Furor Over Gay and Lesbian Studies," in the *Chronicle of Higher Education*, 21 September 1994.

My proposed class, which was approved by my department without dissent, was to cover a variety of topics: differing attitudes toward homosexuality in the Judeo-Christian and Greco-Roman worlds; the history of the gay rights movement; the impact of AIDS on the gay community and the significance of social perceptions of the epidemic as a "gay disease"; gay literature and film; scientific investigations into a "gay gene"; current political battles over such issues as gays in the military, the legalization of same-sex marriages, and antigay legislation.

My motives for proposing the course were similar to those that had inspired me, a few summers earlier, to offer another "Special Topics" class on the Holocaust. Even more than the Holocaust, the subject of homosexuality was completely absent from Montana Tech's standard curriculum. Moreover, to me, both topics highlighted a common theme — the nature and consequences of prejudice. Why are certain minorities stigmatized? What are the results of this stigmatization? How can it be overcome? My Holocaust course had been warmly received, both on and off campus.

> *I am deeply committed to creating in all my classes a forum where students can feel free to express every conceivable opinion, including ones with which I vehemently disagree.*

When I conceived my gay studies class, I was not so naive about the problem of homophobia as not to anticipate some campus gossip and grumbling after the class appeared in the course catalogue. Therefore, I was not shocked when an irate letter from a Tech student surfaced in the student newspaper. "Your . . . intent," the student fumed, "seems bent on persuading people that being gay is a natural thing. . . . What could you possibly study about gays besides their sex lives? You can't put them in the same class with Indians, Hispanics, Whites, and Blacks. . . . What will be the difference between your class and 'The Sally Jessy Raphael Show'? . . . It's pretty sad when an institution with the educational reputation that Tech has will stoop so low as to permit a class to be based on your 'politically correct' agenda." She concluded with a quote from St. Paul's Epistle to the Romans (one I was to be regaled with often in the days ahead) condemning "men with men committing indecent acts and receiving in their own persons the due penalty of their error."

Had it seemed worthwhile, I could have summoned a response to the student's tirade. Why, after all, did she find it so unthinkable, so patently absurd, to equate gays with other persecuted minorities, such as blacks and Native Americans? Why, moreover, should homosexuals be defined exclusively in terms of their sexual practices? Isn't that every bit as dehumanizing as describing heterosexuals solely by the fact that they usually engage in vaginal intercourse? And why, in a democratic society premised on a constitutional separation of church and state, did the letter writer think that merely quoting the New Testament irrefutably clinched her argument — that, in other words, her personal faith had to be obeyed unconditionally by all Americans, regardless of whether or not they shared her beliefs? Most important, what the heck did she have against Sally Jessy Raphael?

Perhaps it was this student, who belonged to the fundamentalist congregation, who informed the pastor of the heresies afoot in the formerly staid precincts of Montana Tech. The pastor's letter to the local newspaper, which sparked the community debate, encapsulated the gay-bashing tactics of the religious right. After praising Tech for its success in training engineers, he reproached it for offering a course in gay studies. While admitting that he was "unclear" as to what the class would actually cover, he warned that "radical homosexuals have an agenda." As proof of such nefarious activity, he quoted a passage allegedly taken from the *Gay Community News*, a weekly Boston newsletter: "We shall sodomize your sons, emblems of your feeble masculinity. . . . They will come to crave and adore us." He lamented the expenditure of tax money on gay studies during a time of cuts in education spending and thunderously concluded: "Our children are important!"

This time I did reply. In my swiftly composed letter, which appeared in the paper two days later, I noted the unfairness of the pastor's insinuation, based on nothing other than the course's title, that my class would promote a "radical homosexual agenda." On the contrary, I insisted that every viewpoint on the issue would be thoughtfully considered. I also pointed out how patronizing it was for the pastor to call college students "children," who should let him decide what they should study. After inviting him to voice his objections to homosexuality in class, I summed up: "To try to censor a course before it has even begun runs contrary. . . to every right a democratic society holds dear."

In retrospect, I think I was right to base my defense of the course on the First Amendment and the principle of academic freedom, rather than on the validity of the gay rights struggle. Not that the decision was easy. The fight for civil rights for gay Americans is a movement I align myself with unequivocally. It was frustrating to have to downplay this commitment in order to deflect charges that my course would be "politically correct." It was no less frustrating to feel obliged, for the same reason, to pledge repeatedly that my class would respectfully consider all points of view — to promise, in other words, to give the homophobes equal time. After all, as my wife mordantly remarked at the time, if I'd taught a course on African-American studies, would I have felt obliged to invite a speaker from the Klan? The analogy is not far-fetched. How much is difference is there, really, between the KKK's view that blacks are subhuman and the Christian Right's official stance that gays are hell-bound sinners and that AIDS is the wrath of God against degenerate sodomites?

On the other hand, as a teacher I am deeply committed to creating in all my classes a forum where students can feel free to express every conceivable opinion, including ones with which I vehemently disagree. Moreover, by focusing on the issue of academic freedom, I was able to rally widespread campus support. As one might expect at a technical school, most of my colleagues are hardly in the vanguard of gay liberation. However, most understood the ominous precedent that would be set if someone unaffiliated with the college could dictate what went on in our classrooms.

Not *everyone*, however. I did receive a letter from a Tech professor, a staunch Baptist, demanding my immediate resignation on the ground that I was morally unfit to be an educator at the college — or, for that matter, at any other school on the planet. Those who "condone, encourage, or participate in gay or lesbian activities," he flatly insisted, "should not be teaching."

Thus, with both the pastor's and my positions publicly staked out and several weeks to go before the class was to begin, the battle was on. A local radio talk show was swamped with calls from listeners who vehemently debated the merits of the class. I missed the program, which was probably just as well, since from what I heard later it sounded about as intellectually substantive as most talk radio. Apparently, most callers insisted that my course should be dropped because it would undoubtedly "recruit" virile heterosexuals to the "homosexual lifestyle." All else aside, such a position implies, of course, that homosexuality is a choice, a notion I've always thought utterly untrue. I wondered how many of those callers ranting about "recruitment" would claim that they personally, if some scheming professor got them in class, could end up persuaded to go to bed with a member of the same sex?

But if their heterosexuality felt like a biological imperative, not a choice, what made them so certain that homosexuals "choose" to be gay?

In contrast to the radio show, the local newspaper ran an admirably balanced front-page story on the controversy. But the dispute was played out most fully in the letters to the editor that deluged the paper for weeks. Here, as before, I received heartening support from my department colleagues. A Tech history professor, for instance, compared the pastor to the Ayatollah Khomeini (which seemed to place me in the unenviable position of Salman Rushdie).

Another colleague, a psychology instructor, explained that, contrary to the pastor's claims, my course wouldn't "waste" tax dollars, since summer classes are self-supporting, with student tuition going to pay instructor salaries. While, practically speaking, this was a key point to clarify, for me it was never the main issue. First off, in our current political climate, allegations of "wasting taxpayer money" are almost never raised in order to further a meaningful discussion about the proper allocation of government funds. Instead, the phrase usually is deployed as a means of mindlessly inflaming the electorate, for whom such terms as "taxes" and "government spending" have been demonized by years of right-wing demagoguery. Such chicanery, I'm convinced, is precisely what the pastor was up to when he raised the issue of taxes.

... several Butte ministers sharply challenged the notion that Christianity is irrefutably anti-gay.

Indeed, had I offered the class during fall or spring semester (when it would have been, in part, taxpayer-funded), I'm convinced it would still have been entirely defensible. The deciding factor for me was not who paid the bills, but whether the class had educational value. As I stated in the local paper, in my view "the major social issues of our time belong in the classroom." Naturally, many Montanans would disagree — especially when the debate moves to a specific subject such as homosexuality. In a conservative state like ours, probably many taxpayers would heartily second the view of one letter writer that teaching a gay studies class is comparable to offering a course on "the ABC's of prostitution or international terrorism." But is it really right to demand that public school teachers merely mirror in class the beliefs of the majority (assuming, of course, that such a consensus can ever be accurately ascertained in our multicultural, politically diverse society), even when those beliefs strike teachers as bigoted and ill-informed? Such an attitude, it seems to me, drags education back into the dark ages.

The dark ages did not, I imagine, produce writing much darker than the pamphlet sent anonymously to every letter writer who supported the course. Issued by an evangelical Christian publisher and blithely titled, "Doom Town: The Story of Sodom," it tells, in comic-book form, of a young Christian who attends a gay rights rally. There, he witnesses gay activists plotting "blood-terrorism" — that is, the poisoning of the nation's blood supply with HIV-tainted blood. Gently pulling aside one of the participants, the Christian relates the story of Sodom. It's an account replete with Biblical drag queens who chase terrified young boys at orgies, while their fellow deviants urge them on by bellowing, "Yeah, fresh meat!" On hearing the tale, the instantly repentant homosexual sobs, "I became a modern day Sodomite because my teachers said it was a harmless alternate lifestyle. . . . Now I'm doomed to hell!" Never fear, his new found friend informs him, there's still hope, for "Jesus can set you free."

. . . when he heard "gay and lesbian" he instantly pictured an activist chanting, "We're queer! We're here! Get used to it!"

Not all the local clergy echoed the sentiments expressed in "Doom Town" and in the pastor's letter. In fact, several Butte ministers sharply challenged the notion that Christianity is irrefutably anti-gay. In the newspaper, a Methodist pastor argued that "strict literalistic interpretations of the Scripture can be injurious, even deadly," and concluded that "science may well discover that homosexuality is as natural and as common a part of human physiology as left-handedness." Another minister, a Congregationalist, wrote, "The Bible has little to say about homosexuality. . . . In contrast, economic . . . injustice [is] mentioned hundreds . . . of times." A second Congregationalist minister insisted that Jesus' core message of love, tolerance, and support for the downtrodden demanded that Christians accept all kinds of people, no matter how different.

With all the backing it received, my class might have withstood the pastor's campaign had he not adopted a second, shrewder strategy — aggressively petitioning the Montana Tech Alumni Association. Mostly mining-industry bigwigs, the alumni soon began besieging Tech administrators with letters and phone calls. They threatened to withdraw thousands of dollars in contributions unless the class was dropped.

The Alumni Association's implacable hostility toward my course (which was completely uninformed, since no alumnus contacted me to learn any specifics about the class) continues to puzzle me. Why, exactly, should a mining executive be so alarmed at the prospect of gay studies at Montana Tech? Why should he even care? Pondering these matters has led me to some admittedly speculative musings. Is there a connection between homophobia and big business? Are the captains of industry, sworn as they are to preserving the status quo, thus pledged by definition to thwarting the aspirations of historically marginalized groups? Is the dog-eat-dog ethos of *laissez faire* capitalism antithetical to a commitment to justice for the oppressed? Is there a tie between the corporate machismo so rife in the business world and the traditional macho revulsion at the perceived effeminacy of gay men? Simply posing these kinds of questions suggests how the field of gay studies, if explored in depth, soon encompasses issues ranging far beyond a narrow focus on homosexuality itself.

It was late on a Friday afternoon, only a few hours before the Alumni Association had scheduled a special meeting to discuss my course, when my division head told me he was canceling the course. Having learned that a local TV-news team was planning to cover the first day of class, he felt that cancellation was in the best interests of the students, who otherwise were at risk of getting caught in the middle of a "media circus." Looking back, I suspect that the reason I didn't challenge his decision was less because I found his rationale defensible (it was, after all, based on the same paternalism toward students that, in my letter, I'd attacked the pastor for exhibiting), than because I was weary of being beleaguered by a controversy that seemed to be escalating out of control.

However, by that evening I knew I'd made an awful mistake. Up to then, all the attacks I suffered had come from without. Now, for the first time, I was pricked by my own conscience, which was infinitely more painful. To live with myself, I knew I had to do all I could to get the course reinstated. That weekend, I telephoned every department colleague I could reach and received their unanimous support — including, surprisingly, that of the division head himself. A kind and decent man, he had, I suspect, grave doubts about his decision all along. Monday morning, he and I met with the academic dean, who agreed to reauthorize the class, asking only that we give it the more innocuous title, "Differing Views on Homosexuality."

Could the whole dispute have been avoided if I'd chosen that title originally? Probably not. Still, the phrase "gay and lesbian" clearly had fanned

127

the flames. One administrator told me that, to him, while the word "homo-sexual" simply connoted someone with atypical sexual desires, when he heard "gay and lesbian" he instantly pictured an activist chanting, "We're queer! We're here! Get used to it!" Perhaps it would have been more politic to have picked this alternate, seemingly neutral title.

On the other hand, as an English professor, I'm well aware that language is never purely neutral. "Homosexual" is a word coined by straights, which not only defines gays exclusively in terms of their sexual practices, but is also historically linked with the belief, once axiomatic in the psychological profession, that homosexuality is a mental illness. In sharp contrast, "gay" is a term gay people have chosen to describe themselves, one whose common usage in gay subcultures actually predates "homosexual" by centuries. Shouldn't a course exploring a minority culture adopt the designation that the culture itself favors? Wouldn't it be obviously racist, say, to title a course on African Americans, "Colored Studies"? Moreover, "gay and lesbian stud-ies" is far less radical than the name currently popular in the humanities: "Queer Studies."

Even with a new, less inflammatory title, the course was still unaccept-able to the college president. He argued that reauthorizing it after the ad-ministration had officially announced its cancellation to the alumni would make the institution look indecisive. Instead, he proposed a compromise: I could "repackage" the class, somewhat shifting its focus while still retain-ing much of its original content, so that it would not appear that the college was reversing its initial decision. The president, the dean, the division head, and I then concocted a "new course," insipidly titled, "Differing Views on Alternative Lifestyles." While still addressing homosexuality, this course also would cover a grab bag of other "non-traditional" lifestyles, including single parenting, living together, and "open" marriages. I regret that by restructur-ing the class this way, we in a sense "closeted" homosexuality by conceal-ing it among a cluster of other "lifestyles." However, because the alternative was losing the class entirely, the president's offer was easy to accept.

Then, not with a bang but a whimper, the dispute faded.

When the paper ran a second front-page story, reporting the replacement of the old class with the new one, the community was informed that the col-lege was not merely capitulating, though I suspect some readers never got

128

past the piece's misleading headline, "Tech Drops Disputed Gay Studies." Still, I was somewhat heartened when the paper printed yet another front-page article, reiterating that the new class would still cover gay issues. That article quoted a fiery press statement from the Butte Human Rights Coalition, which, until then, had focused primarily on fighting the rise of hate groups in Montana. The statement said in part, "We are deeply disturbed by the decision of Montana Tech to cancel the course on gay and lesbian studies. This decision was an act of violence against the community. No weapon was used, but the free exchange of ideas was slain."

As for the pastor who stirred up the whole brouhaha, I've no idea why he chose not to protest my new class as well. Surely, from his perspective, a course that not only studied homosexuality but also lumped in a host of other "sins" could hardly be much of an improvement. Perhaps he concluded that, given all the opposition he'd faced, pressuring Tech into making even a small concession was victory enough. Or maybe he gave up the fight because he was just as worn out as I was.

I find myself viewing the whole affair with some ambivalence, seeing neither victory nor defeat.

Once the uproar died down, and my students and I were allowed to get on with the business of education, the class went fine. Ironically, one positive result of all the controversy was that I had little trouble enlisting a diverse, provocative, and distinguished group of guest speakers. Although the pastor himself declined my invitation to speak, the minister for Tech's Baptist Student Union did take me up on my offer. As staunchly anti-gay as the pastor, she had belonged to the Oregon Citizens' Council that had tried unsuccessfully to pass a ballot measure that would have inscribed the moral condemnation of homosexuality into the state constitution and would have denied gay and lesbian individuals legal protections against discrimination under the pretense of denying them "special rights." She spoke for more than an hour and distributed stacks of literature, making her case lucidly and thoroughly. After she finished, I devoted the second hour to letting students respond with comments and questions.

For all her general savvy, in her opening remarks the minister committed a telling *faux pas* when she mentioned, in passing, how nervous she had been before coming to the class because she feared that students might retaliate by, perhaps, dousing her with HIV-infected blood! This remark, uttered by a bright, educated woman, spoke volumes about the near-clinical paranoia of the religious right. If the only notions one has of gay people are as monsters plotting "blood terrorism," and if, moreover, one sees life as a cosmic struggle between the overwhelming forces of evil and a tiny, beleaguered "elect," such delusions must seem perfectly reasonable.

As a counterpoint to the Baptist minister's talk, I also invited one of the local Congregationalist ministers who had supported the course. She spoke eloquently and at length, also buttressing her argument with numerous Christian references, explaining, among other things, why she was trying to persuade her own congregation to make their church "open and affirming" — which meant welcoming homosexual parishioners and sanctioning same-sex commitment ceremonies. Together, these two sessions presented students with a pair of Christian ministers who drew diametrically opposed conclusions about homosexuality from the same scriptures and similar religious traditions.

Once a religious group enters the political arena, it has no right to call intolerant those who simply disagree with its politics.

Another speaker was a Butte lesbian, who shared her moving life story — one that powerfully dramatized the hardships of growing up gay in small-town America. Trying to deny her sexual orientation, she'd married and had children, which led inevitably to pain and frustration and, finally, a suicide attempt. Later, after she came out, she sought a divorce. But she was denied custody of her children because of her lesbianism. She also was harassed by her neighbors, who vandalized her home, threatened her life, and circulated a petition to have her evicted. Holding her ground, she ultimately won her neighbors' grudging acceptance.

The class also heard remarks by this woman's daughters, now both teenagers and, finally, living with their mother. The girls also had endured years of homophobic taunts, mostly from classmates. With their teased hair and "grunge" attire, they looked like typical American teens, which is just what they were, with the one notable exception that they proved to be as fiercely supportive of gay rights as any activist from ACT UP or Queer Nation. They also were heterosexual. Having a lesbian mother had not "made them gay," although it had certainly made them open-minded.

Perhaps the best presentation of the semester was given by two other out lesbians. One was the executive director of the Montana Human Rights Network, an organization waging a lonely and heroic struggle against the rising tide in Montana of right-wing hate-mongering against gays, Native Americans, Jews, blacks, and women.

The second was the lead plaintiff in a currently pending suit challenging the constitutionality of Montana's anti-sodomy law, a statute similar to laws still on the books in many states that explicitly criminalizes homosexual sexual relations between consenting adults. So far, the state has failed in its attempt to have the suit dropped on the ground that the law is never enforced. While the plaintiffs acknowledge that gay Montanans are not being thrown in jail merely for their bedroom activities, they stress that the law often is invoked to sanction an array of homophobic practices, such as barring gays from the military, denying them child custody, and hindering them in taking legal action when they are victims of discrimination in housing or employment. The law also is a major reason that many Montana homosexuals are afraid to get tested for AIDS, because requesting the test is virtually an admission of criminal behavior. Nor should anyone underestimate the psychic toll wrought by having one's sexuality criminalized by the authorities.

Now that both the furor over the course and the course itself are over, I find myself viewing the whole affair with some ambivalence, seeing neither victory nor defeat. If nothing else, at least the debate broke the community's previously near-total silence on the subject of homosexuality. Even though, like most American towns, no matter how small, Butte has a sizable gay population — a gay bar, a primarily gay theater company, an AIDS support service staffed mostly by gay volunteers — this subculture has remained almost totally closeted. Its low profile is understandable. For example, when a groundbreaking article in the local paper mentioned the founding of a Butte chapter of PFLAG (Parents, Family, and Friends of Lesbians and Gays), the chapter's leader received death threats from Montana's Aryan Nation. Under the circumstances, it's not hard to see why the local "Gay Pride" group convenes at a secret location that changes with every meeting.

Obviously, in this climate, full recognition of Butte's gay population is not going to occur overnight. But after the debate over my class, it now is a bit harder, I suspect, for my neighbors to sustain the fiction that homosexuality is someone else's "problem" or that gays dwell only in big cities. It is also less easy, I believe, for Montana Tech faculty, students, administrators, and alumni to go on thinking that gay studies should exist, if anywhere, only in the ivory towers of Duke or Stanford, surely not at an engineering school in the American West.

So-called political correctness is a complex, ambiguous issue. As I fought to save my class, I began to suspect a hidden agenda behind much of the "anti-P.C." campaign. I concluded that, in my case, the "P.C." label was not an attempt at objective assessment of my course. Rather, the term was being used to club me into silence by dismissively lampooning what I was trying to do. My opponents' main (albeit unstated) objection, I sensed, was not that I was trying to indoctrinate my students or "turn them gay," but simply that I was daring to address the subject of homosexuality in the first place. My critics wanted to shove it back in the closet. Such silencing, of course, is the essence of right-wing "political correctness."

Indeed, the best way to fight the religious right, I've decided, is to stress that the group's underlying ideology is the epitome of right-wing "P.C." — that their theocratic politics clash directly with the democratic principles of individual rights and freedom of speech. In a state college such as Montana Tech, the constitutional separation of church and state applies, just as it does in any other public institution. If church groups can have a gay studies class dropped on the ground that the topic conflicts with Christian doctrine, why not also censor a course on evolution (as has already been done in some public elementary and secondary schools) or comparative religion or existential philosophy — all subjects that, in one way or another, question church teachings?

Perhaps most important, my struggle taught me that no one battling fundamentalism should be silenced by the constant cry of the religious right that its opponents are intolerant of religion — a charge frequently leveled against me during the controversy. Along with noting the hypocrisy of the religious right in labeling anyone else intolerant, progressives should clarify that they are objecting not to the fact that fundamentalist politics are rooted in faith (which is as legitimate a foundation for a political agenda as any other) but rather to the specific political positions espoused in the name of that faith. Once a religious group enters the political arena, it has no right to call intolerant those who simply disagree with its politics.

Finally, liberal educators and politicians need to understand why millions of Americans — especially poor, white, rural Christians — are so susceptible to the homophobic venom of right-wing preachers. Disenfranchised economically, watching their traditional ways of life collapse, many such Americans are looking for someone to blame. Homosexuals often are the scapegoats.

For fellow professors intent on introducing controversial courses, I advise being ready for trouble — especially at tax-supported institutions in the traditionalist American heartland. Had I anticipated the furor that my class would generate, I would have met beforehand with the administration and my department colleagues to develop strategies to combat potential criticism. I would stress that such strategies be assertive rather than defensive, based on staunch adherence to the principle that higher education has a mission to explore all areas of human experience, especially those that have been long suppressed.

Upholding this principle in the midst of battle demands considerable courage, a virtue seldom required in the sheltered groves of academe. But don't we discover the strength of our beliefs only when we are called on to defend them?

Antihomophobic Pedagogy:
Some Suggestions for Teachers*

by Ian Barnard

Despite the current boom in lesbian and gay studies and Queer Theory, most college and university campuses remain hostile environments for lesbian and gay students, staff, and faculty. Lesbian and gay students continue to face formal discrimination in campus housing and benefits policies and informal persecution from homophobic colleagues and teachers and from an institutional apparatus that still excludes lesbians and gay men from its curricula.

Lesbian and gay concerns must not be ghettoized to the pitifully few departments, programs, and courses in Queer Theory and lesbian and gay studies. They must permeate every aspect of every curriculum. I write these suggestions, then, for the teacher who is not teaching a Queer Theory or lesbian and gay studies class, but who nevertheless is committed to the work of decentering heterosexuality in the classroom and in the social realms that the classroom produces and is produced by.

Teaching never can be a neutral activity. The ways we define our disciplines, the texts we teach, the ways in which we teach them, the ways we set up our classrooms, the methods by which we evaluate our students — all

---

*An earlier version of this article appeared in *Radical Teacher* 45 (1994): 26-28. The author thanks the editors of *Radical Teacher* for permission to reprint material here. The author also thanks the following individuals for their assistance: Claire Potter, Janice Chernekoff, Roxana M. Dapper, Henry Abelove, and Molly Rhodes.

these choices (whether our own or not) embody ideological assumptions and have far-reaching effects both inside and outside the classroom. Any anti-homophobic pedagogy will affect all methodologies and epistemologies, both those explicitly concerned with lesbian and gay issues and those that seem to be ignorant of — or even hostile to — some or all lesbian and gay concerns. Whether we teach explicitly lesbian and gay texts or not, whether in fact we have any say over the texts we teach or not, it is in how we read and teach all texts and in how we organize our classrooms and construct our students that we must relentlessly deploy antihomophobic agendas.

1. We should not assume that all our students are straight.

Such an assumption reinforces the invisibility that most lesbians and gay men already suffer. Too often when discussing lesbian and gay issues, even well-meaning teachers (including lesbian and gay teachers) use words like "you," "us," and "them" in a manner that suggests that everyone in the classroom is straight or implies that lesbians and gay men exist only in some comfortably distant place. It is a good idea to remember (and to tell our students) that at least one person in every ten is lesbian or gay. We are almost certain to have at least some lesbians and gay men in our class. And if we are lesbian or gay ourselves, we know for sure that we have at least one lesbian or gay man in the class.

When we ask questions of students or use examples in the classroom, we should not assume that students are heterosexual. Some exercises designed to contest homophobia actually end up re-inscribing it. For instance, role-playing exercises, where students imagine what their world would be like if they were lesbian or gay, or "heterosexual questionnaires," which attempt to undermine the presumption of heterosexual normativity by asking respondents how their heterosexuality was constructed, are great tools for raising heterosexual consciousness. But such activities obliterate the identities of lesbian and gay students in the class. Even such common classroom practices as "freewriting" can be oppressive to lesbian and gay students, for whom truth-telling is not necessarily liberating. (See Hart 1988 and Malinowitz 1992.)

2. We should set an example by not using heterosexist language.

In the classroom, we must avoid examples or language that reinforce many people's assumptions that everyone is heterosexual, that only heterosexuals should be addressed or discussed, or that heterosexuals should be the center of the universe. For instance, rather than saying, "If a woman in a relationship wants to bring her boyfriend to the dance . . . ," we can say, "If a woman in a relationship wants to bring her lover to the dance," or, "If a woman in a relationship wants to bring her girlfriend or boyfriend to the dance."

We also need to tell our students that they should be alert to their own use of heterosexist or homophobic language in their comments in the classroom and in their papers. They should be aware of overtly homophobic language ("all fags should die") and presumptions of universal heterosexuality ("any woman would love to spend a night with Tom Cruise"). We can explain that such language silences the lesbian and gay students in the classroom, who should not be expected to assert or justify their existence.

Often lesbian, gay, and lesbian- and gay-support-ive students will be too frightened to challenge homophobia in a classroom setting.

We also must consistently challenge homophobic stereotypes, assertions, and jokes when students, texts, or other teachers make them. Often lesbian, gay, and lesbian- and gay-supportive students will be too frightened to challenge homophobia in a classroom setting. They rely on us to set an example and to make the classroom a safe environment for them. If we are silent in the face of homophobic comments, we are contributing to the creation of a setting that is personally dangerous and academically unproductive — not only for lesbian and gay students, who might feel directly threatened by these comments, but also for other students who might wish to explore issues around sexuality in their lives or academic work or who are committed to contesting homophobic persecution and discrimination.

3. We should ensure that our students have easy access to addressing lesbian and gay issues, and that students feel that lesbian and gay voices can speak in the classroom.

This means not only including lesbian and gay issues in our discussions, but also using lesbian and gay texts in our courses and inviting papers and projects that present lesbian and gay perspectives and antihomophobic analyses. Students should know that anyone in the class might legitimately write such a paper if they are interested in lesbian and gay issues. Students who choose such topics are not necessarily marking themselves as lesbian or gay.

We also must not assume that students will know that we welcome the discussion of lesbian and gay issues in the class or that we ourselves are antihomophobic and are committed to promoting an antihomophobic classroom environment. Many students still think of lesbian and gay issues as a discussion taboo, and many students will have found that otherwise enlightened teachers are silent, embarrassed, or even hostile when it comes to lesbian and gay concerns. We need, then, to explicitly invite students to address lesbian and gay concerns.

When straight students "come out," the lesbian and gay students are forced to come out to the class, to lie about their sexuality, or to remain silent.

4. We should not make lesbian and gay concerns token elements in our syllabi.

Sometimes teachers want to include lesbian and gay issues in their courses but do so by marginalizing these issues, relegating them to one week in a 15-week course, to one optional reading at the end of the semester, and so on. As a result, students get the message that these issues are not as important as others, that they are an afterthought, or that they are "too controversial" to be included in the main body of the course. Not unexpectedly, then, many students will respond accordingly — with hostility. (See Berg et al. 1989 and Bleich 1989.)

I try to at least say the words, "lesbian," "gay," or "queer," a minimum of once every time I meet with my students, starting with the first day of class. I want to give my students the message that lesbian and gay concerns are a legitimate field of academic inquiry and that lesbian and gay issues will form a central and ongoing concern of our course. If lesbian and gay issues are presented in a non-sensationalistic manner, students usually will respond in kind. I have been surprised to note how quickly my students begin to initiate discussions of lesbian and gay issues and how many of them — of all sexual orientations — choose to write papers and facilitate presentations on lesbian and gay topics once they see that these topics are a legitimate and ongoing theme of the course.

5. We should not base a course on "open-ended" topics, discussions, or texts.

Too often as teachers we feel that we are doing the right thing by assigning our students "open-ended" essay topics or by inviting students to argue "both" sides of a controversial current event. The ideologies and institutions of liberal pluralism tell us that this is the way to promote "free speech" and "democratic" argument. But these kinds of topics and discussions, besides implying that there are only two "sides" to an issue, have the effect of privileging dominant power relations and of further silencing our lesbian and gay students.

For example, if we ask our students to debate whether homosexuality is "wrong" or not, we are expecting our lesbian and gay students to justify their very existence in the classroom — a debate over the rightness or wrongness of heterosexuality would be unthinkable — and to endure painful and threatening homophobic remarks from their colleagues. Lesbian and gay students have a right to expect not to be wounded in this way. Teachers should avoid texts that adopt this type of "pro" and "con" approach (for example, most generic composition readers) and should create assignments that do not invite homophobic responses. Instead of asking students whether homosexuality is "wrong" or not, we might ask them to analyze a homophobic article, explaining who they think the intended audience is, what assumptions the writer makes, what values the argument embodies, and what rhetorical strategies the writer uses.

Better still, we might invite students to analyze, say, Queer Nation's founding manifesto, "I Hate Straights." Instead of asking students to agree or disagree with the article, we could ask them to discuss the article's use of the pronouns "I" and "we." Or we might ask students to conduct some research that could indicate why the article's authors adopt the positions that they do. Or we could invite students to engage with the text as follows: "You are a member of Queer Nation. Explain what you hope to accomplish with this manifesto."

Similarly, students can address such lesbian and gay issues as debates around marriage, monogamy, domestic partnership, and lesbians and gays in the military by treating disagreements *among* lesbians and gay men, rather than generating an inevitable and exclusive binarism between one static homophobic pole and one unified antihomophobic pole.* Thus, instead of arguing whether lesbians and gays should be permitted to marry or not, students can attend to and take positions on the various arguments by lesbians and gay men both for and against marriage. This approach has the advantage not only of encouraging students to work from an antihomophobic position, but also of illustrating the diversity within the lesbian and gay "community" and counteracting many students' stereotypes about a monolithic lesbian/gay experience or a singular "gay opinion" on any given topic.

---

*For examples of articles that could be used for such an assignment, see Friedman (1991) and Job (1993) on lesbians and gays in the military, and Stoddard (1989), Ettelbrick (1989), and Brownworth (1993) on lesbian and gay marriage.

139

The topics that I have suggested are no "narrower" or more "restricted" than any other topics. Every time we give students an assignment, we circumscribe their possible responses. We can choose *how* to circumscribe assignments, not *whether* we should circumscribe them. If teachers do not want to have to read homophobic papers and do not want lesbian and gay students in the class to be subjected to such papers, we have to frame our assignments in ways that do not invite such responses. The best strategy I have found is to ask questions that are genuine questions for us, not ones to which we know the "right" answers. Then not only do students get to participate in a genuine dialogue, but teachers also have the opportunity to learn and grow.

6. We should discourage straight students from "coming out."

Students should realize that when they announce their heterosexuality to the class or preface a comment with the words, "I am straight but . . . ," not only are they (perhaps inadvertently) distancing themselves from lesbian and gay material under discussion instead of engaging with it, but they also are putting the lesbian and gay students in the class in an impossible position. When straight students "come out," the lesbian and gay students are forced to come out to the class, to lie about their sexuality, or to remain silent.

If students do identify themselves as heterosexual, we can ask them why they are making this identification public and invite them to discuss the possible consequences of this public identification for the lesbian and gay students in the class.

Straight teachers also should avoid proclaiming their heterosexuality to the class (either explicitly or by nonchalantly referring to a spouse). In addition to the distancing effect that such a proclamation can have, it has other consequences because of the student-teacher power relation in the classroom. Sometimes such proclamations are made in good faith (a teacher might not want to mislead students or appropriate an identity that he or she feels is not his or her own), but they have the effect of making the classroom a comfortable space for the straight students at the expense of the lesbian and gay students. For example, when lesbian and gay issues or materials are under scrutiny, such a proclamation allows some straight students to breathe a sigh of relief, secure in the knowledge that — despite the sensitivity of the material under discussion — the teacher is "one of us."

Lesbian and gay students might feel that the teacher in this instance is able to discuss queer issues openly only because he or she does so from the safety of his or her announced heterosexuality, a luxury that they do not have. They also are denied the possibility of a role model in the classroom or a point of identification with the teacher. Straight teachers should be willing to run the risk of being thought of as lesbian or gay by their students. They also might want to ask themselves why they choose to identify as straight, especially in light of recent Queer Theory that posits a "queer" identification that does not rely on the same kinds of delimitation of identity that a phrase like "lesbian and gay" might. (Most Queer Theorists have argued that the term "queer" can include some "straights.")

7. Lesbian and gay teachers should come out to students.

Not every lesbian and gay student is a member of a visible campus lesbian or gay group. Some campuses have no such groups. Some students are too afraid to join. Lesbian and gay students — especially those who are not out — sometimes feel isolated and alienated. Given the disproportionately high suicide rate among lesbian and gay teenagers (see Maguen 1991) and the shocking lack of adult lesbian and gay role models for these teenagers, lesbian and gay teachers owe it to themselves and to all their students to be out in the classroom. Lesbian and gay students, including those who are out, need to see real-life, living, institutionally legitimized lesbian and gay professionals standing in front of them, teaching them and their heterosexual peers.

Given the reach of institutionalized homophobia and the relative invisibility of lesbians and gay men in today's society, a lesbian or gay student's or teacher's coming out is not equivalent to a straight student's or teacher's "coming out." In the second case, the power and size of an existing relation of social inequity merely is rehearsed; in the first case, the voice of the "other," just by proclaiming his or her existence, contests that power structure.

Lesbian and gay students . . . need to see real-life, living, institutionally legitimized lesbian and gay professionals standing in front of them, teaching them and their heterosexual peers.

References

Anonymous Queers. "I Hate Straights." *San Diego Gay Times*, 9 August 1990, p. 13.

Berg, Allison, et al. "Breaking the Silence: Sexual Preference in the Composition Classroom." *Feminist Teacher* 4, nos. 2-3 (1989): 29-32.

Bleich, David. "Homophobia and Sexism as Popular Values." *Feminist Teacher* 4, nos. 2-3 (1989): 21-28.

Brownworth, Victoria. "The Matrimonial Noose." *The Advocate,* 19 October 1993, p. 80.

Ettelbrick, Paula L. "Since When Is Marriage a Path to Liberation?" *OUT/LOOK, no.* 6 (1989): 9, 14-17.

Friedman, Mike. "Missing in Action: AIDS, the Military Ban and the 1993 March." *Radical America* 25, no. 1 (1991): 32-37.

Hart, Ellen Louise. "Literacy and the Lesbian/Gay Learner." In *The Lesbian in Front of the Classroom*, edited by Sarah-Hope Parmeter and Irene Reti. Santa Cruz, Calif.: HerBooks, 1988.

Job, Michael. "Gays in the Military: The Choice Is Ours." *Breakthrough* 17 (Spring 1993): 30-34.

Maguen, Shira. "Teen Suicide: The Government's Cover-Up and America's Lost Children." *The Advocate*, 24 September 1991, p. 40-47.

Malinowitz, Harriet. "Construing and Constructing Knowledge as a Lesbian or Gay Student Writer." *PRE/TEXT* 13, nos. 3-4 (1992): 37-52.

Stoddard, Thomas B. "Why Gay People Should Seek the Right to Marry." *OUT/LOOK*, no. 6 (1989): 9-13.

Part Three
Youth, Parents, and Families

Coming Out in the Comics:
A Look at Lynn Johnston's
"For Better or For Worse"

EDITOR'S NOTE: In the spring of 1993, Canadian cartoonist Lynn Johnston created a four-week story about a teenage character named Lawrence. Lawrence was familiar to many readers of Johnston's "For Better or For Worse" comic strip, which appears in newspapers across the United States and Canada. He was well known as a close friend of Michael Patterson, the teenage son in the family on which the strip centers. But "Lawrence's Story" broke new ground, both for the cartoonist and for her readers. Lawrence was gay.

"Lawrence's Story" tells of this teenage boy's struggle to come to grips with his own sexuality. Like many works of fiction, Lawrence's coming out story touches on universal themes. Many gay men and lesbians have faced the same issues and met the same reactions that are portrayed in "Lawrence's Story." And because the story "rings true" for so many gay men, lesbians, their families, and their friends — including the mixing of anguish, denial, isolation, acceptance, and humor — the comic strip is reprinted here with permission from Universal Press Syndicate.

"Lawrence's Story" is included in Lynn Johnston's collection, *"There Goes My Baby!"* (Kansas City: Andrews and McMeel, 1993). In a subsequent collection, *It's the Thought That Counts. . .* (Kansas City: Andrews and McMeel, 1994), Johnston reflected on the story and the reactions that it generated. Telephone calls and faxes poured into the syndicate office and individual newspaper offices across the United States and Canada immediately after the first panel was published. A flood of letters followed. Commented Johnston:

> If I had shown one of the characters shooting another in a school yard, there would have been some reaction, I am certain, but it would have been nothing compared to the controversy started by this story.

However, amid the threats, the curses, the obscenities, and the subscription cancellations, there also arrived what Johnston called the "yes" letters — mail "from doctors, teachers, mental health professionals, clergy, social workers, friends, and families of those about whom the story was written." And, finally, there were responses from gay men and lesbians, letters that Johnston called "direct, honest, and amazingly personal." Wrote Johnston:

> I don't know when I have been so moved. It is not possible to imagine how painful it is to be persecuted and reviled because you are different. These letters were evidence of that.

In the end, more than 70% of the responses turned out to be favorable. But those who have followed Lynn Johnston's comic strip family may sense, as I do, that even if the responses had been overwhelmingly anti-homosexual, Johnston probably would have reached the same conclusion: "My syndicate and many editors allowed me to take a risk. . . and, yes, without question, it was the right thing to do!"

Reader's accustomed to keeping their favorite "For Better or For Worse" panels on the refrigerator may need to buy more magnets. Following is "Lawrence's Story" in its entirety.

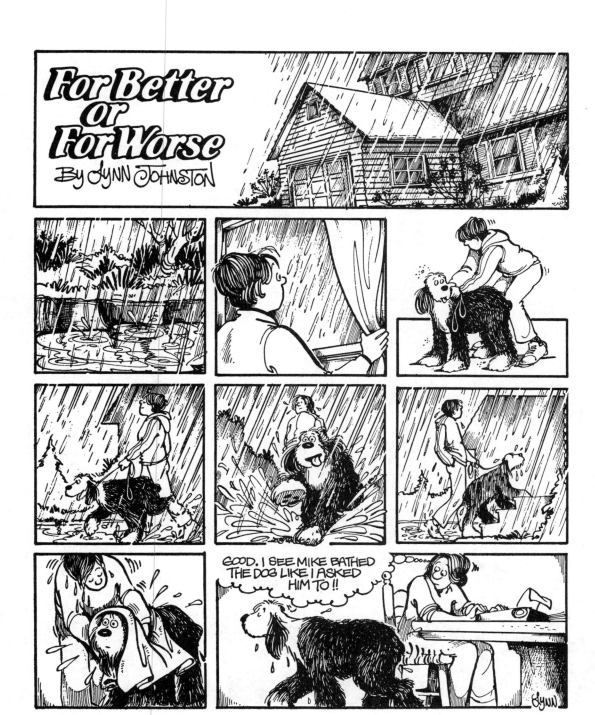

147

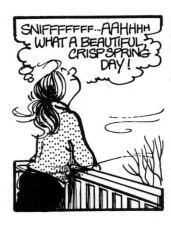

SNIFFFFFFF...AAHHHH WHAT A BEAUTIFUL, CRISP SPRING DAY!

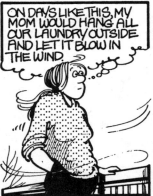

ON DAYS LIKE THIS, MY MOM WOULD HANG ALL OUR LAUNDRY OUTSIDE AND LET IT BLOW IN THE WIND.

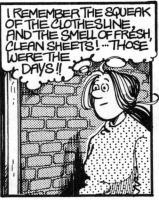

I REMEMBER THE SQUEAK OF THE CLOTHESLINE, AND THE SMELL OF FRESH, CLEAN SHEETS! ...THOSE WERE THE DAYS!!

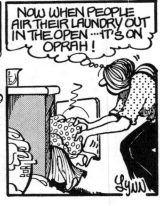

NOW WHEN PEOPLE AIR THEIR LAUNDRY OUT IN THE OPEN ...IT'S ON OPRAH!"

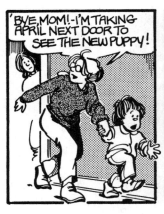

'BYE, MOM!-I'M TAKING APRIL NEXT DOOR TO SEE THE NEW PUPPY!

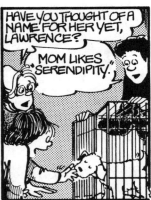

HAVE YOU THOUGHT OF A NAME FOR HER YET, LAWRENCE?

MOM LIKES SERENDIPITY.

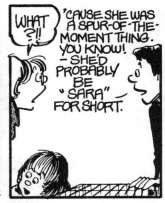

WHAT?!!

'CAUSE SHE WAS A SPUR-OF-THE-MOMENT THING. YOU KNOW! - SHE'D PROBABLY BE "SARA" FOR SHORT.

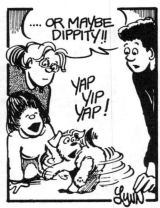

.... OR MAYBE DIPPITY!!

YAP YIP YAP!

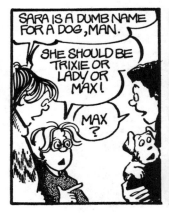

SARA IS A DUMB NAME FOR A DOG, MAN.

SHE SHOULD BE TRIXIE OR LADY OR MAX!

MAX?

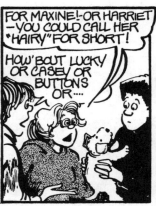

FOR MAXINE!-OR HARRIET - YOU COULD CALL HER "HAIRY" FOR SHORT!

HOW 'BOUT LUCKY OR CASEY OR BUTTONS OR....

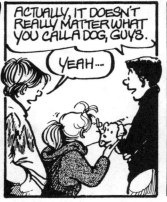

ACTUALLY, IT DOESN'T REALLY MATTER WHAT YOU CALL A DOG, GUYS.

YEAH....

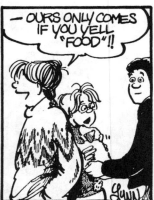

- OURS ONLY COMES IF YOU YELL "FOOD"!!

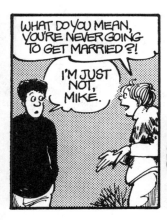

SHRIEK! GIGGLE GIGGLE GIGGLE!

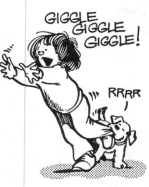

GIGGLE GIGGLE GIGGLE!

RRRR

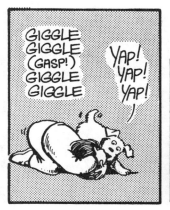

GIGGLE GIGGLE (GASP!) GIGGLE GIGGLE

YAP! YAP! YAP!

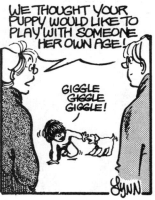

WE THOUGHT YOUR PUPPY WOULD LIKE TO PLAY WITH SOMEONE HER OWN AGE!

GIGGLE GIGGLE GIGGLE!

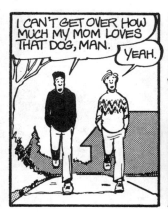

I CAN'T GET OVER HOW MUCH MY MOM LOVES THAT DOG, MAN.

YEAH.

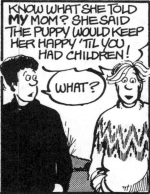

KNOW WHAT SHE TOLD MY MOM? SHE SAID THE PUPPY WOULD KEEP HER HAPPY 'TIL YOU HAD CHILDREN!

WHAT?

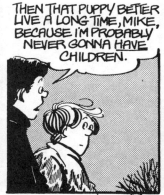

THEN THAT PUPPY BETTER LIVE A LONG TIME, MIKE, BECAUSE I'M PROBABLY NEVER GONNA HAVE CHILDREN.

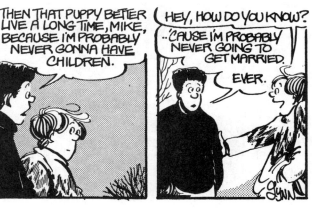

HEY, HOW DO YOU KNOW?

...'CAUSE I'M PROBABLY NEVER GOING TO GET MARRIED. EVER.

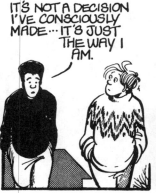

WHAT DO YOU MEAN, YOU'RE NEVER GOING TO GET MARRIED?!

I'M JUST NOT, MIKE.

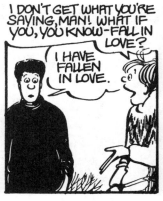

IT'S NOT A DECISION I'VE CONSCIOUSLY MADE... IT'S JUST THE WAY I AM.

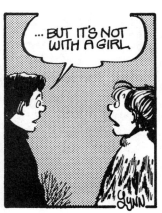

I DON'T GET WHAT YOU'RE SAYING, MAN! WHAT IF YOU, YOU KNOW—FALL IN LOVE?

I HAVE FALLEN IN LOVE.

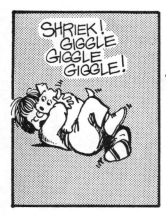

...BUT IT'S NOT WITH A GIRL.

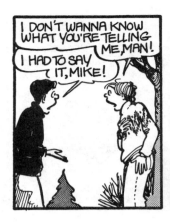

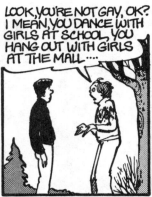

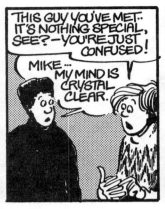

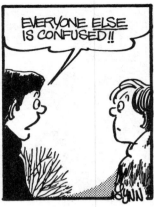

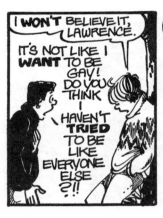

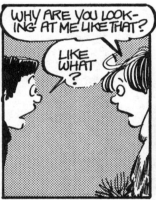

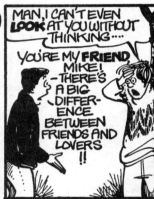

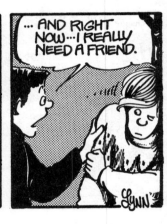

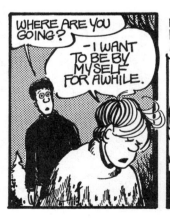

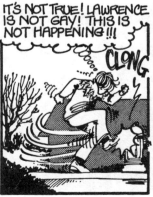

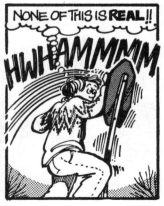

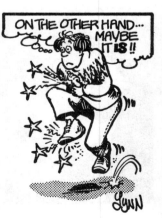

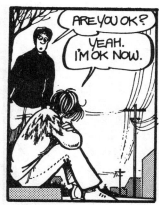

ARE YOU OK?

YEAH. I'M OK NOW.

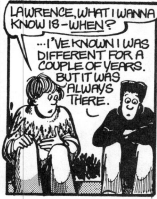

LAWRENCE, WHAT I WANNA KNOW IS—WHEN?

...I'VE KNOWN I WAS DIFFERENT FOR A COUPLE OF YEARS. BUT IT WAS ALWAYS THERE.

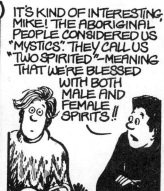

IT'S KIND OF INTERESTING, MIKE! THE ABORIGINAL PEOPLE CONSIDERED US "MYSTICS". THEY CALL US "TWO SPIRITED"—MEANING THAT WE'RE BLESSED WITH BOTH MALE AND FEMALE SPIRITS!!

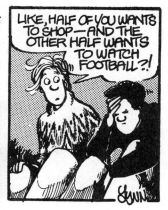

LIKE, HALF OF YOU WANTS TO SHOP—AND THE OTHER HALF WANTS TO WATCH FOOTBALL?!

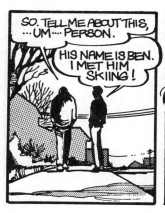

SO. TELL ME ABOUT THIS, ...UM....PERSON.

HIS NAME IS BEN. I MET HIM SKIING!

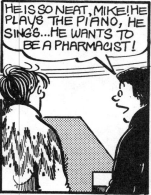

HE IS SO NEAT, MIKE! HE PLAYS THE PIANO, HE SINGS...HE WANTS TO BE A PHARMACIST!

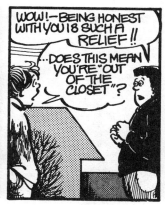

WOW!—BEING HONEST WITH YOU IS SUCH A RELIEF!!

...DOES THIS MEAN YOU'RE "OUT OF THE CLOSET"?

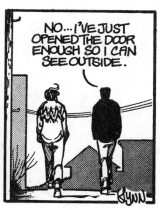

NO...I'VE JUST OPENED THE DOOR ENOUGH SO I CAN SEE OUTSIDE.

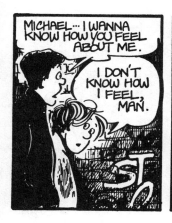

MICHAEL...I WANNA KNOW HOW YOU FEEL ABOUT ME.

I DON'T KNOW HOW I FEEL, MAN.

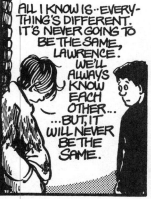

ALL I KNOW IS...EVERYTHING'S DIFFERENT. IT'S NEVER GOING TO BE THE SAME, LAWRENCE. WE'LL ALWAYS KNOW EACH OTHER... ...BUT, IT WILL NEVER BE THE SAME.

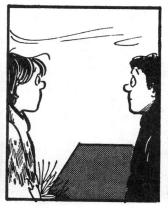

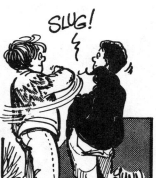

SLUG!

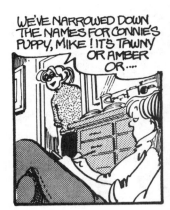

WE'VE NARROWED DOWN THE NAMES FOR CONNIE'S PUPPY, MIKE! IT'S TAWNY OR AMBER OR...

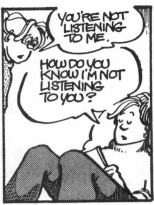

YOU'RE NOT LISTENING TO ME.

HOW DO YOU KNOW I'M NOT LISTENING TO YOU?

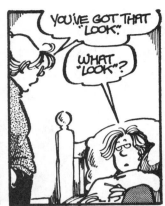

YOU'VE GOT THAT "LOOK."

WHAT "LOOK"?

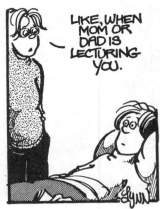

LIKE, WHEN MOM OR DAD IS LECTURING YOU.

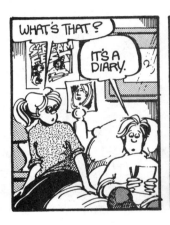

WHAT'S THAT?

IT'S A DIARY.

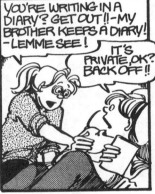

YOU'RE WRITING IN A DIARY? GET OUT!! — MY BROTHER KEEPS A DIARY! — LEMME SEE!

IT'S PRIVATE, OK? BACK OFF!!

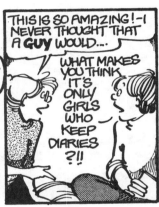

THIS IS SO AMAZING! — I NEVER THOUGHT THAT A **GUY** WOULD...

WHAT MAKES YOU THINK IT'S ONLY GIRLS WHO KEEP DIARIES?!!

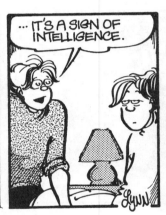

... IT'S A SIGN OF INTELLIGENCE.

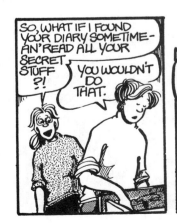

SO, WHAT IF I FOUND YOUR DIARY SOMETIME — AN' READ ALL YOUR SECRET STUFF?!

YOU WOULDN'T DO THAT.

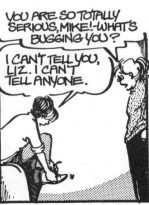

YOU ARE SO TOTALLY SERIOUS, MIKE! — WHAT'S BUGGING YOU?

I CAN'T TELL YOU, LIZ. I CAN'T TELL ANYONE.

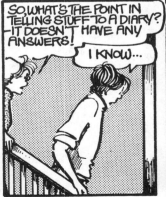

SO, WHAT'S THE POINT IN TELLING STUFF TO A DIARY? IT DOESN'T HAVE ANY ANSWERS!

I KNOW...

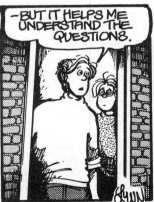

— BUT IT HELPS ME UNDERSTAND THE QUESTIONS.

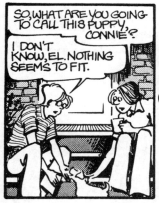

SO, WHAT ARE YOU GOING TO CALL THIS PUPPY, CONNIE?

I DON'T KNOW, EL. NOTHING SEEMS TO FIT.

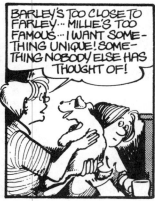

BARLEY'S TOO CLOSE TO FARLEY... MILLIE'S TOO FAMOUS... I WANT SOMETHING UNIQUE! SOMETHING NOBODY ELSE HAS THOUGHT OF!

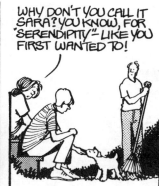

WHY DON'T YOU CALL IT SARA? YOU KNOW, FOR "SERENDIPITY"- LIKE YOU FIRST WANTED TO!

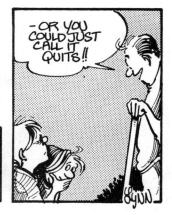

-OR YOU COULD JUST CALL IT QUITS!!

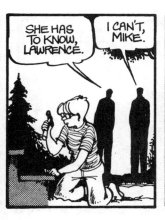

SHE HAS TO KNOW, LAWRENCE.

I CAN'T, MIKE.

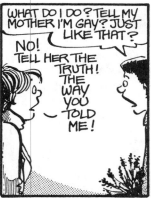

WHAT DO I DO? TELL MY MOTHER I'M GAY? JUST LIKE THAT?

NO! TELL HER THE TRUTH! THE WAY YOU TOLD ME!

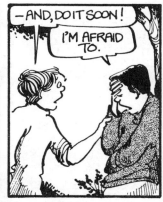

-AND, DO IT SOON!

I'M AFRAID TO.

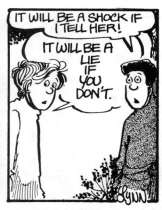

IT WILL BE A SHOCK IF I TELL HER!

IT WILL BE A LIE IF YOU DON'T.

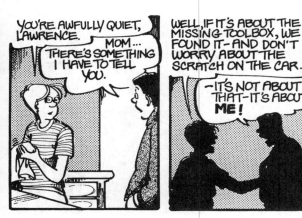

YOU'RE AWFULLY QUIET, LAWRENCE.

MOM... THERE'S SOMETHING I HAVE TO TELL YOU.

WELL, IF IT'S ABOUT THE MISSING TOOLBOX, WE FOUND IT- AND DON'T WORRY ABOUT THE SCRATCH ON THE CAR...

-IT'S NOT ABOUT THAT-IT'S ABOUT ME!

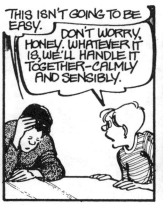

THIS ISN'T GOING TO BE EASY.

DON'T WORRY, HONEY. WHATEVER IT IS, WE'LL HANDLE IT TOGETHER-CALMLY AND SENSIBLY.

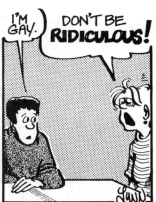

I'M GAY.

DON'T BE RIDICULOUS!

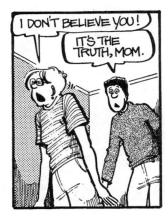

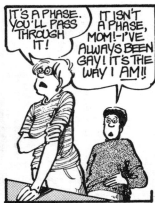

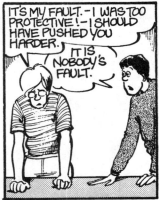

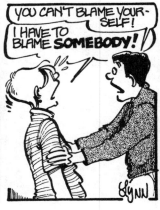

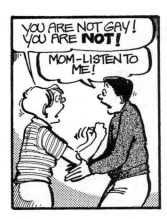

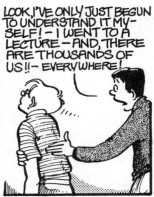

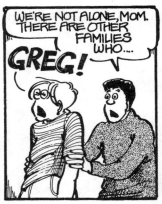

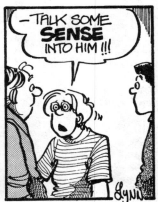

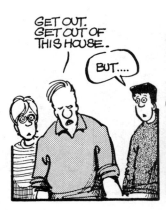

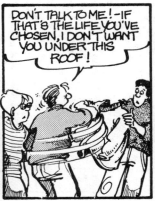

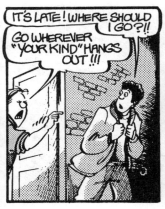

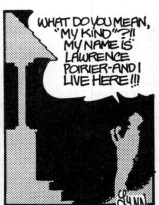

154

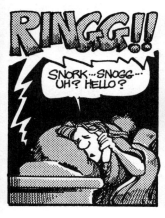

RINGG!!

SNORK...SNOGG... UH? HELLO?

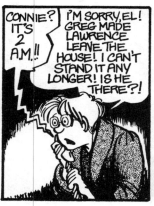

CONNIE? IT'S 2 A.M.!!

I'M SORRY, EL! GREG MADE LAWRENCE LEAVE THE HOUSE! I CAN'T STAND IT ANY LONGER! IS HE THERE?!

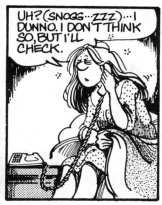

UH? (SNOGG...ZZZ)...I DUNNO. I DON'T THINK SO, BUT I'LL CHECK.

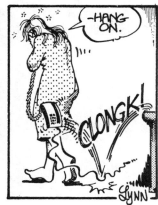

—HANG ON.

CLONGK!

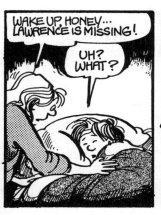

WAKE UP HONEY... LAWRENCE IS MISSING!

UH? WHAT?

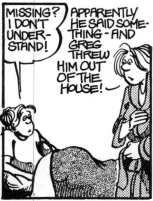

MISSING? I DON'T UNDERSTAND!

APPARENTLY HE SAID SOMETHING - AND GREG THREW HIM OUT OF THE HOUSE!

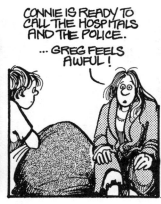

CONNIE IS READY TO CALL THE HOSPITALS AND THE POLICE.

...GREG FEELS AWFUL!

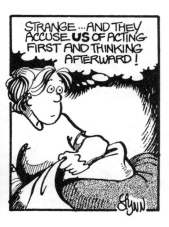

STRANGE...AND THEY ACCUSE **US** OF ACTING FIRST AND THINKING AFTERWARD!

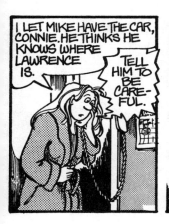

I LET MIKE HAVE THE CAR, CONNIE. HE THINKS HE KNOWS WHERE LAWRENCE IS.

TELL HIM TO BE CAREFUL.

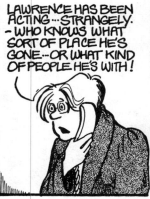

LAWRENCE HAS BEEN ACTING...STRANGELY. - WHO KNOWS WHAT SORT OF PLACE HE'S GONE...OR WHAT KIND OF PEOPLE HE'S WITH!

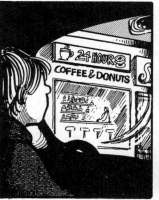

24 HOURS
COFFEE & DONUTS

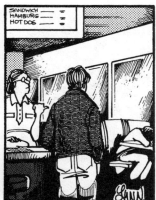

SANDWICH
HAMBURG
HOT DOG

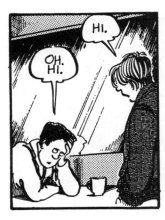

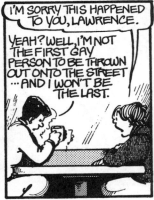

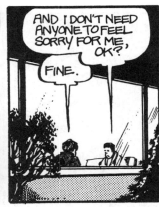

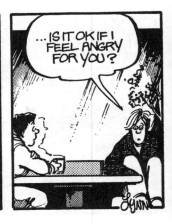

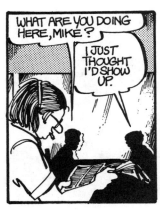

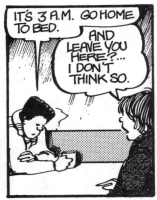

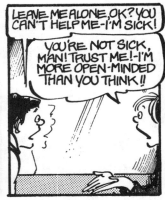

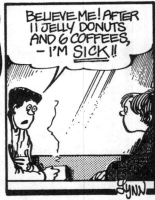

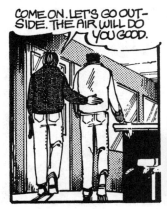

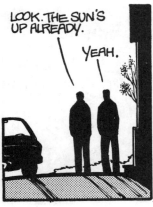

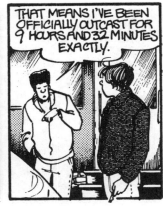

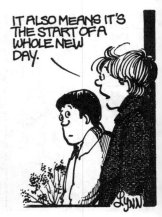

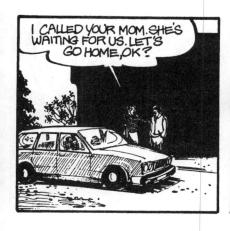

I CALLED YOUR MOM. SHE'S WAITING FOR US. LET'S GO HOME, OK?

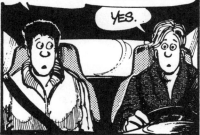

MIKE.. REMEMBER WHEN YOU SAID THAT NOTHING WOULD EVER BE THE SAME BETWEEN US... THAT WE'D PROBABLY ALWAYS KNOW EACH OTHER — BUT THAT'S ALL?

YES.

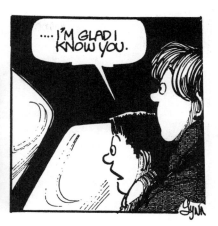

.... I'M GLAD I KNOW YOU.

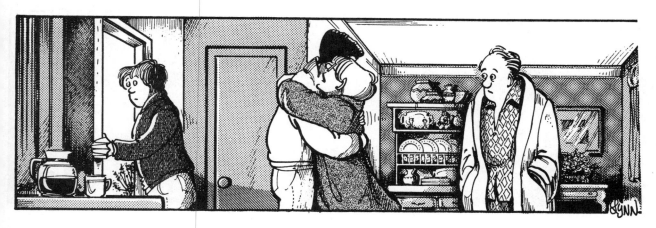

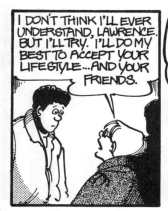

I DON'T THINK I'LL EVER UNDERSTAND, LAWRENCE. BUT I'LL TRY. I'LL DO MY BEST TO ACCEPT YOUR LIFESTYLE...AND YOUR FRIENDS.

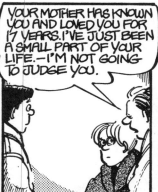

YOUR MOTHER HAS KNOWN YOU AND LOVED YOU FOR 17 YEARS. I'VE JUST BEEN A SMALL PART OF YOUR LIFE. — I'M NOT GOING TO JUDGE YOU.

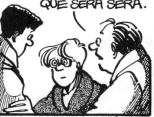

AS LONG AS YOU'RE A GOOD MAN.... AND A KIND MAN - I'LL RESPECT YOU.

... AS FOR THE REST.. WHAT WILL BE WILL BE. QUE SERA SERA.

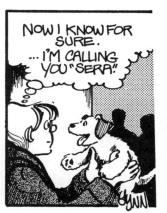

NOW I KNOW FOR SURE. ... I'M CALLING YOU "SERA."

Were You Born with the Lifestyle You Chose?

by David Timothy Aveline and Kathryn Brown

This article provides an analysis of 1,120 questions about homosexuality collected for gay/lesbian/bisexual speaker panels. These questions, collected from students at a Midwestern university for discussion at gay/lesbian/ bisexual (GLB) speaker panels, are sorted into categories and analyzed on two levels: 1) subject matter of questions and 2) underlying attitudes and values that the questions imply.

At the first level, 12 categories emerged covering a variety of subjects. At the second level, three themes emerged: 1) GLB people as curiosities, 2) pressures GLB people face in society, and 3) GLB people as threats to the conventional social order.

Homosexuality is an increasingly controversial topic that evokes strong opinions as to its rightful place in society. After more than a decade of AIDS, well-publicized struggles for gay rights in social and political arenas, and major initiatives to outlaw the "promotion of the homosexual lifestyle" in states such as Oregon and Colorado, it is difficult not to know of large communities of gays, lesbians, and bisexuals. GLB people also have been frequent guests on television talk shows, characters in major Hollywood movies, and the center of a national debate over their exclusion from military service.

In spite of this heightened public exposure — and in spite of the questions many people might have about GLB people as a result — there has been a noticeable lack of education on homosexuality in high schools and universities (Sears 1991). Unless students take courses in human sexuality, abnormal psychology, or deviant behavior, they may well go from their freshman to senior college years with no substantial mention of GLB issues. Even then, such courses often treat homosexuality as a special case, set apart from mainstream concerns, and restricted to a single lecture.

In short, public discourse on GLB issues has increased while education lags behind. Consequently, when young people are exposed to such issues, they often interpret them on the basis of beliefs long disproven by science, yet stubbornly held in place by silence, ignorance, and intolerance.

College campuses are not only centers for learning, but arenas for moral and ideological debate, places where solid friendships are formed, and diverse environments where young people come of age. For these reasons, young GLB people often are visibly out of the closet, filled with new-found pride and vitality, and vocal about who they are and what they believe. Many colleges now have politically active GLB student organizations, gay dances, and annual pride rallies. Some even witness occasional "kiss ins," openly gay or lesbian couples living in campus housing, and even gay fraternities. For many students, such occurrences are likely their first real exposure to GLB people and GLB concerns. Before they came to college, homosexuality might easily have been dismissed as something to joke about or condemn. But when faced with real GLB people — open, vocal, and unashamed — they may be puzzled. What is homosexuality? Where does it come from? Why do those people "flaunt it"?

One way to answer such questions on university campuses is through GLB speaker panels, typically used in sociology, psychology, and education courses. Course instructors invite groups of gays, lesbians, and bisexuals, usually students themselves, to talk about their experiences growing up, coming out, and dealing with harassment and hostility. (For a description of GLB speaker panel implementation, see Croteau and Kusek 1992.) The result often is a productive dialogue between panel members and students, where direct questions are asked and answered, correct information is given, and fears are allayed. Much research now exists to testify that education in general on issues pertaining to homosexuality is effective in combating homophobia (Anderson 1981; Curtis and Heritage 1991; Goldberg 1982; Iyriboz and Carter 1986; Stevenson and Gajarsky 1990; Wells 1989) and that GLB speaker panels in particular are effective means of such education (Chng and Moore 1991; Green, Dixon, and Gold-Neil 1993; Lance 1987, 1992; Morin 1974; Pagtolun-An and Clair 1986).

As educators at a large Midwestern university, we have been conducting GLB speaker panels for several years. They have been positively received and, while no formal measurement has yet been undertaken, we believe highly successful in dispelling myths and reducing hostility. As one sophomore majoring in sociology who attended a panel said, "This is the first time I've seen gay people. They're nothing like the stories I heard back home."

"Were you born with it or did you decide to be gay?"

But not all students speak up so easily. Because of shyness, fear of peer disapproval, or similar reasons, the vast majority who attend speaker panels are silent. To compensate for this, we began to ask instructors to collect written questions from students several days before a panel was scheduled, and panel members responded to them during their presentation. It is these questions — of which we now have 1,120 — that we address in this paper.

By definition, a question is a request for specific information. But, taken further, it also reflects a number of qualities about the asker with respect to the matter under inquiry, such as level of knowledge, level of confusion, values, past experience, underlying concerns, and so on. Therefore, an analysis of any set of questions reveals not only what the askers want to know but also the information they already hold and how they regard that information. For example, those who ask if homosexuality is caused by inherent traits or environment are requesting an "either-or" statement as to its cause. But by their very inquiry, they reveal a preoccupation with cause and, in turn, a particular belief system about sexual normality. They may even reveal some degree of confusion in this respect in *how* they ask the question, as suggested by the title of this paper, "Were You Born with the Lifestyle You Chose?"

A number of books have been published that provide answers to the most frequently asked questions about homosexuality (for example, Marcus 1993). At least one systematic study of such questions has been conducted (McCord and Herzog 1991). But to our knowledge, no research has done more than categorize the questions or answer them. In our analysis, we attempt to go further. We ask not only what questions are being asked, but what they reveal about the knowledge, concerns, and values of those who ask them.

Method

"Did your parents freak out when you told them?"

Our original database was a cardboard box filled to the brim with more than a thousand pieces of paper. Some were crumpled, others were folded, and still others were mere scraps torn roughly from school notebooks. Some were bundled with elastics and marked with a course name and number; others lay loose, tumbled on top of one another with no marked origin. Each had a question printed or hurriedly scribbled on it, and some had two or three questions. These questions were collected by instructors for scheduled speaker-panel presentations in sociology, psychology, education, and nursing courses. They represented at least nine semesters.

Our first task was to organize the questions. We entered them, as they were written, into a database and assigned each question a number. Only two questions were illegible and had to be discarded. The final count was 1,163 questions. Next, we sorted the questions into categories according to the various themes that emerged. This process yielded 37 categories, which we later collapsed into 13. Finally, for purposes of this analysis, we chose to omit one category — Pedagogical Concerns (for example, "What can I do as a future teacher do to help gay students?") — because that category was specific to a single profession. Thus the final sample comprised 1,120 questions sorted into 12 categories. These categories are summarized in the following section.

Results

Cause/Nature: (n=230, 20.5%) This largest category included not only concerns about cause and nature, but also how many GLB people there were in society and whether people could change their sexual orientation. Virtually all of these questions can be reduced to two underlying themes: What is homosexuality? and Where does it come from?

Of those concerned with cause, nearly half asked whether homosexuality can be attributed to biology or individual choice (for example, "Were you born with it or did you decide to be gay?"). Others tried to pinpoint some traumatic occurrence that they suspected somehow triggered a homosexual orientation, such as a bad childhood, early experimentation with the same sex, a bad relationship with the opposite sex, and an overly affectionate mother. One student wanted to know if homosexuality resulted from excessive masturbation, believing this to be the reason most religions forbade it. Still others wanted to know if panel members were homosexual or bisexual out of rebellion or a desire to shock.

Questions about nature accounted for 28% of the questions in this category. The modal question was, "What attracts you to the same sex?" Others wanted to know if homosexuality is similar to heterosexuality, if panel members hated opposite-sex members, or what makes people know they are homosexual or bisexual. Most questions about bisexuality concerned which sex bisexual panel members preferred, why they are "dissatisfied" with only one sex, and if they told their opposite-sex sex partners of their bisexuality.

As for the remaining questions, some concerned sexual orientation change — whether panel members were attracted to the opposite sex previously or would be in the future. Others wanted to know about "male and female roles" in homosexual relationships. And a few wanted to know if the number of GLB people is increasing because of media publicity.

Coming Out, Realization, Acceptance: (n=160, 14.3%) These questions pertained to panel members' formative experiences as GLB people. Here, the question most often asked was, "When did you first realize that you were gay (lesbian or bisexual)?" Students who asked this were not necessarily concerned with a specific age as much as they were with a stage in life when homosexual or bisexual feelings emerge. Coming out questions similarly concerned a life period, and the remaining questions concerned degree of difficulty in panel members' accepting themselves as GLB people in society.

Prejudice, Discrimination, Harassment: (n=115, 10.3%) Most questions here dealt with whether panel members had been victims of prejudice, discrimination, or harassment, or details concerning such treatment (for example, "Have you ever had people hassle you because you're gay?"). Ten students asked about outright gay bashing and 10 more asked about discrimination in the work place. The remainder asked how panel members reacted to, handled, or felt about homophobic people or negative treatment.

Openness, Outness, Actions in Public: (n=113, 10.1%) These questions all dealt with whether panel members readily told others about their sexual orientation, if they engaged in public displays of affection, or why some GLB people "flaunted" themselves in front of others. Many of these questions implied that such openness hurts the "gay cause," is disgusting, or at the least is unnecessary because heterosexuals do not flaunt their sexuality.

Family, Friends: (n=96, 9.6%) This category dealt with whether parents or friends know of panel members' sexual orientations, how the panel members told others of their sexual orientation, and what reactions they received. Most asked about parents, others asked about friends, and still others asked about siblings or grandparents. Implicit in the vast majority of these questions was the assumption that a gay, lesbian, or bisexual son or daughter would be difficult for parents to accept (for example, "Did your parents freak out when you told them?"). A few questions further implied that this would be even more difficult for a same-sex parent.

Religion, Morality: (n=78, 7%) The majority of religious questions concerned panel members' religiosity or religious beliefs, their rationales toward Judeo-Christian proscriptions against homosexuality, or whether the panel members thought themselves wrong or sinful. Some students quoted specific biblical passages (for example, Leviticus 18:22) in their questions, and a few wrote wholly condemning statements (for example, "Opposite sex is the right normal Godly way!").

Relationships, Dating, Boundaries: (n=72, 6.4%) While some of these questions concerned relationship status or desired qualities in partners, the majority had two underlying themes: 1) whether panel members were able to identify other GLB people before approaching them (for example, "How can you tell if someone you want to date is gay?"), and 2) whether they cross sexual orientation boundaries by "hitting on" or having relationships with heterosexuals (for example, "Would you hit on a straight person to try and change him?"). The remainder of questions in this category concerned locales or techniques for meeting other GLB people.

Child Rearing, Gay Parenthood: (n=65, 5.8%) Two themes emerged here: whether GLB people should be parents and whether panel members wanted to raise children in the future. Implicit in many of the former questions was that same-sex parents would somehow confuse children (for example, "How would a child learn his proper role with two mommies?"), and implicit in many of the latter was that GLB people would be missing out on one of life's more joyful experiences.

HIV/AIDS, Sexuality: (n=61, 5.5%) Considering that homosexuality is commonly associated with AIDS in much societal discourse, surprisingly few questions broached this subject. Most questions in this category dealt with panel members' first sexual experiences or the kinds of sex acts that two men or two women typically perform. Some students implied that any same-sex sexual encounter at an early age "hooks" people on homosexuality and that they would have been heterosexual otherwise. Those wanting to know about actual sex practices most often asked about anal intercourse.

Support, Community: (n=36, 3.3%) Two types of questions were placed in this category: whether GLB people had resources they could rely on for social and emotional support and the extent of the GLB community on campus or in town. A few further asked how they, as heterosexuals, could be supportive.

Teenage Homosexuality: (n=23, 2.1%) Questions about younger GLB people covered a range of areas. Implicit in some questions was an underlying belief that homosexuality is wrong for teenagers and that they should be discouraged from having sex. Other questions dealt with obstacles GLB teens might face. One student asked about harassment in high school, another asked about suicide rates, and still another asked about support networks.

Miscellaneous: (n=71, 6.3%) This catch-all category was reserved for all questions not fitting into other categories. Students here asked about popular music personalities, whether homosexuals make up a "race," if homosexuality is contagious to children, if panel members cross-dressed, and so on.

"Are gay teens really gay or just confused?"

Discussion

Before looking at the data in greater depth, we point out two of their limitations. First, since the questions were not gathered randomly and are restricted to a single Midwestern university campus, they are in no way generalizable to the greater population; nor are they representative of all college students. However, they are useful because they illustrate a variety of concerns and give clues to students' underlying knowledge, values, and attitudes toward homosexuality. This, rather than strict measurement of attitude

165

distributions among populations, is where the value of the data lies, and it is the thrust of our analysis.

Second, the questions have no information about their askers that might otherwise have been valuable in discerning attitude differences by race, age, size of city of permanent residence, religion, and sex. For example, there is now much research among college students to suggest that males are less tolerant of GLB people (Herek 1988; Kite 1992; Kunkel and Temple 1992; Larson, Reed, and Hoffman 1980) and that acceptance of homosexuality is inversely related to religiosity (Hong 1983, 1984; Irwin and Thompson 1977; Maret 1984; Seltzer 1992). More research is needed on the relationship of questions on homosexuality to such variables.

To reiterate our main premise, an analysis of any set of questions takes place on two levels. First, one addresses what is asked as an indicator of what kind of information the asker wishes to know. Second, at a deeper level, one addresses how and why something is asked, which ultimately gives clues to the asker's underlying belief system. A question is not only a request for specific information, it is both a reflection of a specific concern and an indicator of a specific attitude. What is asked is as significant as what is answered, and how a question is asked ultimately suggests something about the asker's beliefs with respect to the matter at hand. In this sense, the 1,120 questions reveal some substantial areas of misinformation and discomfort about homosexuality, most of which can be reduced to three major themes: 1) GLB people as curiosities, 2) pressures GLB people face in society, and 3) whether homosexuality will impose itself on the conventional heterosexual order. We will look at each separately.

GLB People as Curiosities. As Adam (1982) suggested, while American society has become increasingly pluralistic in terms of race, religion, and ethnicity, it continues to resist sexual pluralism. As a result, homosexuality continues to be a mystery, an oddity, and a curiosity. A great many questions dealt with the cause of homosexuality, its nature, when people come to realize their sexual orientation, whether a first homosexual experience makes one a homosexual, and what same-sex couples do with each other sexually. Simply stated, these questions seem to be: What is it? Where does it come from? Why does it exist?

These concerns come as no surprise considering the continued deviant status of GLB people, the importance of opposite-sex dating in adolescent and young adult life, and the predominance of Judeo-Christian values in American society, particularly with regard to marriage and family. In a society where love and sex are defined primarily as heterosexual, those oriented toward the same sex become enigmatic. This is evident in a renewed interest in the search for essentialist causes of homosexuality. Recent research in this area has revolved around size differentials in the hypothalamus and genetic predispositions (Byne and Parsons 1993; Pool 1993). It also is evident in the emergence of a number of grassroots organizations, such as Love in Action, Desert Stream Ministries, and Exodus International, which offer to "cure" GLB people through religious ministration. Such discourse — saying ultimately that homosexuality should not exist — has very likely permeated students' general attitudes. As a result, GLB people continue to be seen as curiosities.

Pressures GLB People Face in Society. Being a curiosity is not without costs. The questions on coming out, self-acceptance, prejudice and discrimination, family and friends, and teenage homosexuality all show a strong awareness among students that GLB people face considerable obstacles in society. These questions related to what students saw as inevitable difficulties that GLB people have or will face at some point in their lives: Parents are likely to disapprove; longtime friends may abandon them; many people may harass them; they may be denied employment; and they may struggle to come to terms with their own identities.

Ironically, many students saw these difficulties as reciprocal. While most questions dealt with GLB people's own difficulties, some implied that they, by their nature, impose hardships on others. This was especially evident in questions about parental acceptance that were phrased in ways such as, "Was your father *disappointed* when you told him?" or "Did your parents *blame* themselves for very long?" Implicit here is that a sense of failure, sadness, and disappointment are natural parental reactions to having a GLB child.

Questions on teenage homosexuality carried with them a great deal of concern that GLB teenagers may feel isolated in a world where few resources exist for them and a belief that "kids can be cruel" to people who are in some way different. We suspect that many who asked about GLB teens recalled their own recent experiences growing up and imagined how those around them might have reacted (or perhaps did react) in high school to GLB class-mates. Even so, there was an underlying sentiment — illustrated by such questions as "Are there any signs of teenage homosexuality?" and "Are gay teens really gay or just confused?" — that homosexuality is wrong for teen-agers or that swift and efficient intervention could steer them onto a hetero-sexual path.

GLB People as Threats to the Conventional Social Order. As an argument against homosexuality, it often is said that if it were the only state in exis-tence, the population would die out. Christian fundamentalist rhetoric further suggests that homosexuality threatens to undermine the American family and, as a result, will weaken the nation as a whole (for example, Fein and D'Souza 1993). A substantial proportion of the questions carry similar im-plications: that homosexuality is functionally threatening to heterosexuality and that it exists in direct opposition to the family and the conventional social order.

Clues to this perceived threat can be seen in questions about bisexuality. While few questions dealt directly with this subject, many that did expressed fears that bisexuals might have an opposite-sex relationship while secretly engaging in same-sex affairs. In this respect, they illustrate a fear that homo-sexuality, with all of its perceived dangers, will seep into and disrupt a het-erosexual world.

Homosexuality may be seen as threatening by some students, but they may further see it as separate and, thus, self-contained. Bisexuality, on the other hand, represents a point of juncture between the homosexual and heterosex-ual worlds and so, among other things, an implied link to HIV infection. If some heterosexual students perceive themselves as invulnerable to AIDS, believing that not being in a "high-risk group" somehow exempts them (see Gelman et al. 1987), then bisexuality threatens to bring HIV infection over an implied boundary and is thus threatening in itself.

Many questions on relationships, dating, and homosexual-heterosexual boundaries also implied a fear of homosexual infiltration. While some ques-tions concerned relationship qualities, dating rituals, and how GLB people find each other, others dealt with whether GLB people (gay men in particu-lar) try to "recruit" heterosexuals or, at the very least, attempt to seduce them.

One student asked if gay men "acted like women" to attract heterosexual men; another asked if gay men looked for young boys because they are impressionable; and still another asked if lesbians try to steal men's girlfriends. Similarly, many questions were phrased in familiar rhetoric that asserts that any mention of homosexuality is an attempt to encourage a homosexual lifestyle (for example, York 1988). One student asked if "recruitment" of heterosexuals was part of the "homosexual agenda." Implicit in these questions is a belief that homosexuality is perpetuated through seduction, promotion, and aggressive "marketing."

Conclusion

On the first level of analysis — what is asked — the questions reveal that students were concerned about a wide variety of issues in regard to GLB people and homosexuality. These concerns alone show that education would be beneficial in transferring desired information to college students in general. But, on the second level — how and why something is asked — the questions reveal substantial areas of bias, misinformation, and fears, which strongly suggest that information transfer alone is inadequate. Education is more than the simple transfer of information on demand; to do so is to assume that those demanding the information are fully aware of what is important. On the contrary, and at least in cases of such emotionally charged issues as homosexuality, education must make people aware of their own attitudes, how they are formed, and how those attitudes shape their thoughts. To address the question of whether homosexuality is biologically rooted or societally induced accomplishes only half the task. It is necessary to look at why the question is asked to begin with.

References

Adam, B.D. "Where Gay People Come From." *Christopher Street* 6 (1982): 50-53.
Anderson, C.L. "The Effect of a Workshop on Attitudes of Female Nursing Students Toward Male Homosexuality." *Journal of Homosexuality* 7 (1981): 7-69.
Byne, W., and Parsons, B. "Human Sexual Orientation: The Biologic Theories Reappraised." *Archives of General Psychiatry* 50, no. 3 (1993): 228-39.

Chng, C.L., and Moore, A. "Can Attitudes of College Students Toward AIDS and Homosexuality Be Changed in Six Weeks? The Effects of a Gay Panel." *Health Values* 1, no. 2 (1991): 41-49.

Croteau, J.M., and Kusek, M.T. "Gay and Lesbian Speaker Panels: Implementation and Research." *Journal of Counseling and Development* 70, no. 3 (1992): 396-401.

Curtis, D.E., and Heritage, J. "Influencing Homonegative Attitudes in College Students Through an Educational Unit on Homosexuality." Paper presented at the Annual Meeting of the Middle Tennessee Psychological Association, Nashville, 1991.

Fein, B., and D'Souza, D. "Society Should Not Sanction Gay Partnerships." In *Homosexuality: Opposing Viewpoints*, edited by D. Bender and B. Leone. San Diego: Greenhaven Press, 1993.

Gelman, D.; Drew, L.; Hager, M.; Anderson, M.; Raine, G.; and Hutchison, S. "A Perilous Double Life." *Newsweek*, 13 July 1987, pp. 44-46.

Goldberg, R. "Attitude Change Among College Students Toward Homosexuality." *Journal of American College Health* 30, no. 6 (1982): 260-68.

Green, S.; Dixon, P.; and Gold-Neil, V. "The Effects of a Gay/Lesbian Panel Discussion on College Student Attitudes Toward Gay Men, Lesbians, and Persons with AIDS (PWAS)." *Journal of Sex Education and Therapy* 19, no. 1 (1993): 47-63.

Herek, G.M. "Heterosexuals' Attitudes Toward Lesbians and Gay Men: Correlates and Gender Differences." *Journal of Sex Research* 25 (1988): 451-77.

Hong, S.M. "Sex, Religion, and Factor Analytically Derived Attitudes Towards Homosexuality." *Australian Journal of Sex, Marriage, and Family* 4 (1983): 142-50.

Hong, S.M. "Australian Attitudes Towards Homosexuality: A Comparison with College Students." *Journal of Psychology* 117 (1984): 89-95.

Irwin, P., and Thompson, N.L. "Acceptance of the Rights of Homosexuals: A Social Profile." *Journal of Homosexuality* 3 (1977): 107-21.

Iyriboz, Y., and Carter, J.A. "Attitudes of a Southern University Human Sexuality Class Toward Sexual Variance, Abortion, and Homosexuality." *College Student Journal* 20, no. 1 (1986): 89-93.

Kite, M.E. "Individual Differences in Males' Reactions to Gay Males and Lesbians." *Journal of Applied Social Psychology* 22 (1992): 1222-39.

Kunkel, L.E., and Temple, L.L. "Attitudes Towards AIDS and Homosexuals: Gender, Marital Status, and Religion." *Journal of Applied Social Psychology* 22 (1992): 1030-40.

Lance, L.M. "The Effects of Interaction with Gay Persons on Attitudes Toward Homosexuality." *Human Relations* 40 (1987): 329-36.

Lance, L.M. "Changes in Homophobic Views as Related to Interaction with Gay Persons: A Study in the Reduction of Tensions." *International Journal of Group Tensions* 22 (1992): 291-99.

Larson, K.S.; Reed, M.; and Hoffman, S. "Attitudes of Heterosexuals Toward Homosexuality: A Likert-Type Scale and Construct Validity." *Journal of Sex Research* 16 (1980): 245-57.

Marcus, E. *Is It a Choice?* San Francisco: HarperCollins, 1993.

Maret, S.M. "Attitudes of Fundamentalists Toward Homosexuality." *Psychological Reports* 55, no. 1 (1984): 205-206.

McCord, D.M., and Herzog, H.A. "What Undergraduates Want to Know About Homosexuality." *Teaching of Psychology* 18, no. 4 (1991): 243-44.

Morin, S.F. "Educational Programs as a Means of Changing Attitudes Toward Gay People." *Homosexual Counseling Journal* 1 (1974): 160-65.

Pagtolun-An, I.G., and Clair, J.M. "An Experimental Study of Attitudes Toward Homosexuals." *Deviant Behavior* 7, no. 2 (1986): 121-23.

Pool, R. "Evidence for Homosexuality Gene." *Science* (1993): 261, 291-92.

Sears, J.T. "Helping Students Understand and Accept Sexual Diversity." *Educational Leadership* 49 (1991): 4-6.

Seltzer, R. "The Social Location of Those Holding Antihomosexual Attitudes." *Sex Roles* 26 (1992): 391-98.

Stevenson, M.R., and Gajarsky, W.M. "Issues of Gender in Promoting Tolerance for Homosexuality." *Journal of Psychology and Human Sexuality* 3, no. 2 (1990): 1-163.

Wells, J.W. "Teaching About Gay and Lesbian Sexual and Affectional Orientation Using Explicit Films to Reduce Homophobia." *Journal of Humanistic Education and Development* 28 (1989): 18-34.

York, F. "Does Your Public School Promote Homosexuality?" *Focus on the Family Citizen* 12 (June 1988): 6-8.

Gay Youth in the Family*

by Jill Gover

Adolescence is an important period of development that involves the integration of biological, psychological, and social demands. During adolescence, lesbian and gay youth often become aware of their sexual orientation. Adolescents' problems do not stem from their sexual orientation per se, but from the hatred that is directed at them because of their orientation. Internalization of this hatred intensifies their problems and contributes to self-destructive behavior. Without support from their families, many lesbian and gay adolescents are unable to cope with the unique stressors that a homophobic society creates. Fear of rejection by family members creates tremendous anxiety in young gay people. This intense stress is aggravated by isolation and a sense of difference.

Rejection by Family

Many parents believe the myths regarding the role of parents in the development of homosexuality. They mistakenly believe that their role modeling determines whether or not a child will grow up lesbian or gay. Numerous studies have refuted this myth as nonscientific and unsubstantiated; nevertheless, many parents still believe that they've done something wrong when their child discloses a homosexual orientation. Parental reactions can include

*This essay first appeared in the *Journal of Emotional and Behavioral Problems* (Winter 1993). Reprinted with permission of the author.

denial, anger, guilt, insistence on therapy to "change" the young person, and sometimes abuse and expulsion from the home.

The continuing lack of family support creates many problems for lesbian and gay youngsters and interferes with their emotional and cognitive development. Rejection by family is a major stressor contributing to suicidal behavior. Conflict with family members regarding sexual orientation increases the young person's sense of not belonging, which further lowers self-esteem. Many adolescents who disclose their sexual orientation to their family are rejected, mistreated, or become the focus of the family's dysfunction. Sometimes the rejection is so severe that it leads to violence. When the violence occurs within the family, running away or expulsion from the home is frequently the result. These "throwaway kids" often end up on the streets involved in prostitution or "survival sex" and are at risk for contracting HIV/AIDS.

Goffman points out that "passing" divides the stigmatized into two groups: the discredited and the discreditable (1963). The discredited are those whose stigma is known or visible. Those whose stigma is hidden or unknown, but for whom discovery would be disastrous, are discreditable.

Gay people who are "discredited" because they've been "discovered" face reactions ranging from humiliation to violence. Nina, a 15-year-old, had tremendous difficulty struggling with the rejection she faced at home because she was an "out" lesbian. Pressure to change her outward appearance, fights with her parents over girlfriends, verbal threats of violence, and ultimately a rape, triggered a severe depressive episode.

Hidden homosexually oriented adolescents see what happens to the "discredited" and fear that the same thing might happen to them, which intensifies their fear of discovery and creates severe stress. They feel compelled to maintain their "discreditable" position, living with a deep, dark, shameful secret.

Isolation

This isolation prevents access to accurate information for gay and lesbian adolescents. Lack of information is not limited to absence of information; even more damaging are the misinformation and unbelievable antilocutions promulgated in our culture and reinforced in the home. The most deleterious effect of such misinformation on a naive, developing adolescent is a cognitive dissonance that will adversely affect the young person's sense of self.

There is little or no opportunity for homosexually oriented adolescents to discover what it means to be homosexual. They are unique among minorities in that they do not share minority status with their family of origin. An African-American child might face harassment and rejection in a racist society, but at least he or she experiences love and acceptance in the home that ameliorates the negative effects of racism. Gay adolescents often lack positive role models and the community support necessary to develop a positive self-image. Therefore, they cannot envision or sometimes even conceive of a future for themselves that is not based on shame.

The cognitive isolation perpetuates a hopeless, helpless, worthless triad of core beliefs that is the cornerstone of depression (Beck 1967). When misinformation is pervasive and accurate information or positive gay role models are inaccessible, the shame intensifies, frequently leading to self-destructive behavior.

Because many gay young people are afraid to disclose their sexual orientation to their parents, siblings, or friends, they often feel emotionally isolated. In a survey of clients at the Institute for the Protection of Lesbian and Gay Youth in New York City, 95% of the clients interviewed expressed feelings of being alone, of being the only one who feels this way, of having no one to share feelings with. They wanted to be able to talk with someone gay, especially an adult gay person, outside of a sexual context. A young gay man wrote this about his emotional isolation:

> Why can't we say where we are really hurting? . . . I was convinced that the only way I could be accepted was to remain hidden. I was sure that no one would love me if they knew. . . . I was desperate. I couldn't continue. I withdrew from school and almost killed myself.

Emotional isolation leads to clinical depression. Gay youth who are emotionally isolated experience pervasive loss of pleasure, feelings of overwhelming sadness, changes of appetite, sleep disturbances, slowing of thought, lowered self-esteem, and strong feelings of shame and failure. They repeatedly report that they feel alone in the world, that no one else is like

There is little or no opportunity for homosexually oriented adolescents to discover what it means to be homosexual.

them, and that they have no one to whom they can confide or talk freely. A young lesbian expressed this feeling in her journal:

> In October I realized my lesbianism and I did not have someone to talk with. I recall the anguish I suffered looking back over my journal during that time period. Please help me. . . . I have to talk with someone. . . . I have to tell someone, ask someone. WHO? . . . Would someone please help me? Someone, anyone. Help me. I'm going to kill myself if they don't.

Social and emotional isolation are significant factors in adolescent promiscuity, especially among gay males.

A developmental task of adolescence is individuation and separation from family. Nevertheless, family still has primary importance. In a survey administered by the Maryland state government, an overwhelming majority of the high school students sampled wished that their parents would spend more time talking with them. Adolescents experience an emotional tug-of-war, wanting to be independent yet still needing the nurturance and guidance of parents. They want to act like adults, but they still need the acceptance, love, and guidance of parents. Despite the stereotype of the "acting out" rebellious teenager, many teens still turn to parents for help when faced with difficult decisions, anxiety, or stress.

Gay teens are no different. Parents who accept their children's gay sexual orientation find that the issues of parenting remain the same. It doesn't matter whether 16-year-old Jane dates Sue or Jim when it comes to curfew, time on the phone, car privileges, homework, and all the other aspects of living with a teenager. Once the shameful secret is "out of the closet" and family members are supportive, gay adolescents are less likely to develop emotional and behavioral disorders. For example, gay parents who have gay children often report that their kids are "typical teenagers"; they struggle with the same parent/teen conflicts facing all parents of adolescents.

However, most gay teens do not come from gay households. Typically they grow up in a world that at best ignores them. Early on, they sense they are different; and they interpret that difference negatively. Adolescence is a time of conformity and the formation of sexual identity. For gay youth, the experience of difference comes from the conflict between the gender identity and role expected by family and society and the person's inner sense of gender

176

identity and role. John, a quiet 19-year-old, wrote the following about his experience of feeling different from his peers:

> When I was in grade school and junior high, I had lots of friends and I had a great time. But when I started high school my friends. . . began to relate to each other in a different way. The guys started talking about girls and getting turned on. . . . I realized that I wasn't interested in the girls that way, and I was concerned. Then I began to realize that I was becoming more interested in the guys — that I was thinking about them in the same way they were talking about girls. I wondered what was going on — if I was inadequate, if I was O.K. I was pretty anxious, but there wasn't anybody to talk to. I used to stand around with the guys and try to look interested in all their gas about this girl and that so I wouldn't be alone. . . . All the time I'd be thinking about one or the other of them. It seemed like I didn't belong. . . . I was on such a bummer with myself, I'm not sure what would have happened if I hadn't met . . . , before I lost self-respect totally.

Social and emotional isolation are significant factors in adolescent promiscuity, especially among gay males. Isolated socially from other gay people and emotionally starved, these vulnerable teens learn to make "contact" in certain neighborhoods, bookstores, movies, parks, etc. Unfortunately, this contact is solely sexual in nature. The casual sex maintains the "discreditable" position, as it compartmentalizes and separates sex from other aspects of one's life. Moreover, the intensity of sexual feelings that accompany these clandestine encounters are easily mistaken for romantic love by gay adolescent males. When their "love" is unrequited, they may feel unable to get their intimacy needs met and lose hope that they will ever sustain a relationship.

The setting, the danger, and the type of individuals who exploit young people in this way all tend to reinforce the belief that homosexuality is bad and shameful and that homosexuals are sick people. This exacerbates an already negative self-image and further isolates the teens. When they hear the same negative messages at home about homosexuality, they come to believe that they are worthless human beings and do not deserve to live. Heterosexual teens are able to discuss their romances and break-ups with family members and friends, but a homosexual teen keeps all those feelings inside, which intensifies the pain, grief, and loss.

Ethnic minority youth constitute a significant percentage of teens who identify as gay, lesbian, bisexual, or transsexual. Gayle Porter, program director of the Child and Family Therapy Center at St. Elizabeth's Hospital in Washington, D.C., estimates that at least one million of America's gay youth are African 84

American, and about 750,000 are Hispanic.

Ruth Hughes, coordinator of gay youth services at the Center for Special Problems in San Francisco, reports that minority gay youth experience more severe social and cultural oppression than other gay youth and much more serious problems than other adolescents. Ethnic minority youth face all of the psychosocial stressors that other gay youth face and, in addition, are confronted with the economic discrimination, prejudice, and oppression facing minorities. They are subjected to stressors created by homophobia *and* racism.

African-American gay youth have a particularly difficult time. They frequently are discriminated against by white homosexuals and often ostracized by their own ethnic group because of their sexual orientation.

Two issues that strongly affect ethnic minority youth are religion and family. Many ethnic minorities belong to religions that view homosexuality as a sin. Ethnic minority gay youth internalize these strong religious messages and believe they will go to hell for their sins. Many ethnic minority families see their gay children as an embarrassment to their cultural group and view homosexuality as disrespectful to the family and God. Ethnic minority youth have a tremendous fear of being rejected by their families, which is exacerbated by the isolation they already feel in this society as people of color. For these youths, rejection by family is a major risk factor for suicide.

Interventions

Specific interventions can reduce the risk of emotional and behavioral problems and strengthen the internal resources of gay youth. First, a conscious effort must be made to promote homosexual role models at all levels of society. Most people agree that it is important to have positive role models for minority students, but many gay and lesbian professionals, teachers especially, are still "in the closet," afraid of adverse consequences if they are open about their sexual orientation. Moreover, the very subject of gay youth creates feelings of fear in some homosexual caregivers. Gay mental health professionals fear that if they work with gay youth as "out" homosexuals, they will be accused of recruiting and lose their license to practice. In a needs assessment of a mental health agency by Robinson and Martin (1983), 61% of the respondents feared negative reactions if they openly addressed the problems of gay youth.

Despite these obstacles, there are innovative educational programs and services for gay youth. Project 10 in Los Angeles and the Harvey Milk School in Manhattan are two models designed to meet the needs of gay and lesbian teens.

Positive role models are critical for dispelling myths and creating hope . . .

Project 10 began in 1985 as a dropout prevention program at Fairfax High School. It was developed by a high school teacher, Virginia Uribe, who saw that a high percentage of gay and lesbian students was dropping out of school. The project now is run by the Los Angeles Unified School District and has evolved into a flexible model with four components: education, school safety, dropout prevention strategies, and counseling services. The program invokes responsibility of heterosexual society to all its members, however diverse. Educational components include a speaker's bureau of gay/lesbian youth, training and consciousness-raising for school staff, and the inclusion of positive gay material in the school library. In addition, policy requires school authorities to report and respond immediately to all anti-gay incidents of harassment and violence. However, the key component of this program is counseling. Informal discussion groups, drop-in individual counseling, and peer counseling are available for gay, lesbian, bisexual, transgender, and questioning youth. The opportunity to meet in a safe space with peers and supportive adults breaks the isolation that is so devastating to gay youth.

Critical to the success of Project 10 has been the collaboration with social service agencies in Los Angeles. The Los Angeles Gay and Lesbian Community Services Center has a Youth Services Department that offers seven weekly youth discussion groups; a hotline, called Youth Talkline, that is designed to reach isolated gay youth; and an emergency shelter for homeless, "throwaway" gay young people. Gay and Lesbian Adolescent Social Services provides two group homes and foster placements for gay youth rejected by their families. Gay-sensitive job training, mental health, and medical services are now available to gay youth in Los Angeles, all of which counteract isolation, homophobic attitudes, and a negative self-image. Project 10 is an example of community-based, integrated, school-linked services for a high-risk population; and its success lies in the key components of education, counseling, and support services.

The Harvey Milk School opened in 1985 as part of the Institute for the Protection of Gay and Lesbian Youth. The school opened because many gay youth were not succeeding in the New York City public schools. Whether lesbian and gay youth were open about their identities or not, societal prejudice took its toll; and many students were antisocial, abusing alcohol and other drugs, depressed, or suicidal. The school is one of many alternative schools in Manhattan designed to serve as a transitional program with the intention of mainstreaming students back into traditional schools. Counselors and teachers assist students in acquiring coping skills and positive self-esteem through focus groups, individual counseling, peer counseling, and role-playing. The goal is to help these students process the traumas they've endured in the past and build confidence and support to prepare for the future. The school is small — 24 students, mostly between the ages of 15 and 17 — offering a traditional academic curriculum, but also providing substantial social services, including a family counseling program to assist family members in accepting the student's sexual orientation.

Interventions that provide information, acceptance, and support are necessary in order for gay teens to overcome the psychosocial stressors they confront growing up in a homophobic society. We must promote family acceptance and understanding of gay youth if we are to reduce their risk of dropping out of school, substance abuse, suicide, and other life-threatening behaviors.

Interventions that provide education and support for families are critical. Parents need to be educated about the nature and development of homosexuality. They need to know that homosexuality is another healthy form of sexual expression and that they are not to blame for anything wrong. Although we do not know what causes homosexuality, any more than we know what causes heterosexuality, parents should be aware of recent research that indicates a predisposition in some people toward a particular sexual orientation, which limits the role of family in its development. Parents need to understand the powerful impact they have on their children's self-esteem. They need to be encouraged to communicate to their gay child that he or she is still loved and cared for as an individual, regardless of sexual orientation.

In order to break through the cognitive isolation of gay youth, schools need to take responsibility for educating all students about homosexuality. Curricula, library books, and media resources should include information relevant to gay youth. As accurate information is more readily accessible to all students, gay youth will be less likely to internalize self-deprecating stereotypes and falsehoods about homosexuality. Instead, they will learn about adult gay role models who have made significant contributions to society.

Schools also need to protect gay youth from abuse by peers and to provide them with a safe environment in which to learn. A strong disciplinary policy should be implemented and enforced on those who victimize gay students.

Counseling services are extremely important in order to provide emotional support and ameliorate depression. Alternative programs need to be available for those who cannot succeed in the traditional school setting. These interventions in the schools would do a lot to enhance resiliency and decrease destructive behavior among gay youth.

Gay youth also need access to peer support and recreational activities in order to reduce their isolation and enhance positive social development. Positive role models are critical for dispelling myths and creating hope and vision for the future. In the absence of family support, caring adults may be the lifeline for a gay adolescent struggling to find his or her place in the world.

Last, but certainly not least, professional counseling and social services for gay youth are critical interventions.

Mental health professionals need specialized training on issues pertinent to gay youth. Suicidality needs to be explored with youth who identify as gay, and psychosocial stressors need to be assessed in relation to a homosexual orientation. The goal of treatment is to assist sexual minority youth in developing a positive self-image and to support them as they confront conflicts associated with their sexual orientation.

Gay youth face a hostile environment, rejection from loved ones, and isolation. The traumatic consequences of these psychosocial stressors make homosexually oriented teens more vulnerable to substance abuse, chronic depression, and other self-destructive behaviors. Acceptance, care, and concern by family members is instrumental in creating a buffer for these vulnerable youth.

References

Beck, A. *Cognitive Therapy and the Emotional Disorders*. New York: Harper & Row, 1967.

Bell, A., and Weinberg, M. *Homosexualities: A Study of Diversity Among Men and Women*. New York: Simon & Schuster, 1978.

Bernard, B. *Resiliency and Protective Factors*. Far West Laboratory Regional Center, 1990.

Clinical Psychiatry News. New Orleans: International Medical News Group, July 1991.

Gibson, P. *Report of the Secretary's Task Force on Youth Suicide*. U.S. Department of Health and Human Services, 1989.

Goffman, E. *Stigma: Notes on the Management of Spoiled Identity*. Englewood Cliffs, N.J.: Prentice-Hall, 1963.

National Gay Task Force. *Anti-Gay/Lesbian Victimization: A Study by the National Gay Task Force in Cooperation with Gay and Lesbian Organizations in Eight U.S. Cities*. New York, 1984.

Old Enough to Know

by Shulamit Kleinerman

One rainy afternoon I cut my Spanish class at Phillips Academy and holed up in my room to write an anonymous letter to a gay student I'd never met. The only out student I knew of, Stephen intrigued me because he was so outspoken and seemed so sure of himself, defying student convention with his pastel suits and fluctuating hair color. On my second day at school as a ninth-grader, I'd seen him camp up an orientation skit: "Hi, I'm Stephen, your new roommate. Can I be on top? In the bunkbeds, I mean." When I began to accept my own homosexuality near the end of that school year, I wrote to Stephen, needing some sort of response to my confusion. How could I *know* I was a lesbian? I wasn't asking for advice from an all-comprehending authority. What I needed was the response of an equal.

Stephen passed the letter on to a friend who wrote back, giving his own frank opinions on the many issues I brought up. Responding to my mention of my mother's lesbianism, he wrote, "I'm rather jealous. . . at least you'll have guaranteed support from one corner." His assumption that a gay parent would support the coming-out process of a gay daughter seemed logical, as any gay person has been through a similar process at some point. But when I came out to my mother, she said, "So, you think you're a lesbian," justifying her dubiousness with, "Well, you're rather young to know that."

I was 15 at that time. I had first concretely questioned my sexuality at 13; I could remember wondering at my homosexual feelings (though at the time I was unable to clearly define them as such) at least as far back as the age of five. This was not a whim. Still, again, when a close friend of mine mentioned my homosexuality to her father, he asked, "Is she sure? She could be wrong." Neither my mother nor my friend's father were questioning the validity of homosexuality — they both know better, especially my mother. But they were, rather patronizingly, denying my ability to understand myself, basing their judgment solely on my age.

I had first concretely questioned my sexuality at 13.

While my lesbian mother's response may seem strange, I have received similar reactions from other gay adults. A member of a gay speakers' bureau told a group at my school, "We gay people can be just like you," assuming the heterosexuality of the student audience and failing to acknowledge that several of its teenage members might be (indeed were) gay or bi. I once listened to a lesbian prep-school teacher discuss the circumstances under which she would "allow" a hypothetical same-sex student relationship to continue in her dorm, telling us flatly what was "age-appropriate." Soon after I told my mother I was a lesbian, my mother said, "Well, all right, as long as you don't shave your head. . . ," as though my sexual identity were a symptom of the latest adolescent fashion trend.

Lucky for me, she grew to understand that I did not need or want patronizing adult appraisals. Since then, I have welcomed her support. What gay youth do need is to be accepted into the ranks of lesbian, bi, and gay people as full-fledged members. Our needs and our experiences as gay people differ little from those of adult homosexuals and bisexuals. Being teenagers does not shelter us, for example, from the pain of discrimination. When my roommate's parents withdrew her from our dorm against her will, they were motivated by homophobia directed in equal measure at me and at the lesbian faculty member living on our floor. From experience, we all know that homophobia does not distinguish its victims by age. Our positive counterbalance to the negativity of prejudice must embrace both old and young. Youth does not dilute sexuality.

Just as teenagers are no less gay than the adults that surround them, many of us also are no less deserving of the respect automatically accorded our elders. If the yardstick for maturity measures self-awareness and a comprehension of the surrounding world, then nothing ushers us into adulthood better than coming out. We look into ourselves for an understanding of our sexuality and its importance in our lives, and then we affirm our presence by coming out amid the daunting onslaughts of homophobia, even if just to one person. This courageous process often solidifies identity and world view, providing "adult" stability, regardless of one's age. Gay adults should remember this truth from their own experiences; the soul-searching that accompanies a young man's coming out at 14 is very likely the same process that boosted a now-graying lesbian into adulthood 30 years ago.

In this soul-searching, perhaps we achieve a certain advantage over many of our straight peers. Since they have been conditioned to believe that theirs is the "normal" sexual preference, they need not give their heterosexuality another thought. Meanwhile, gay adolescents become aware of society's heterosexist dominance. Realizing that we had to make an issue out of "accepting" our sexuality because we'd been taught to assume we were straight, we must question why this conditioning exists. How is it unwittingly perpetrated? Facing homophobia in the media, in our schools, from our parents and friends, we must decide if and how to respond. If we are able to fight it, are there ethical issues involved in how we do so? Unable to take our sexuality for granted, we often bring a much more critical eye to the world than an adolescent is usually given credit for. While our straight classmates may simply accept what they have always heard, we must face the "adult" task of creating our own value system. Coming out often is coming of age.

Of course, youth groups and similar "safe spaces" somewhat separate from adults do provide necessary support while this process occurs. When I wrote my letter to Stephen, I was tapping into an informal student support network. Transferring to another school, Northfield Mt. Hermon, the next year, I met a bisexual senior who became a sort of "big brother" to me. It is important that we find the support of others facing the same challenges, especially while we are so often overlooked by adults.

However, once gay students have taken advantage of this peer support, we find ourselves on the front lines of gay visibility. Schools increasingly are becoming a battleground for gay rights. When homophobes claim that teenagers are too young to discuss "abnormal" sexualities, we counter them by something so normal as bringing a date to the prom. And even more important is our effect on fellow students. In the adolescent quarantine that high school imposes, we are chipping away at the homophobia of peers who, not long from now, will enter the adult workplaces where our elders still question our convictions. Those of us lucky enough to be able to publicly come

Coming out often is coming of age.

out can directly challenge prejudice by refusing to remain silent. As a group, gay youth make a valid contribution to the education of their generation, keeping in mind that today's students are tomorrow's leaders and workers. Gay students are worthy of adults' respect.

After all, isn't this the same kind of respect sought from the public by the gay rights movement itself? Homosexuality often is considered acceptable but less desirable and less important than heterosexuality. Similarly, teenagers' opinions and concerns may be heard by adults but relegated to second-class status in favor of the "wiser" views of adults. This is ageist condescension. Like our culture's homophobia, it says, in effect, that we must be confused, or that perhaps, poor things, we are victims of our families' mistakes. Perhaps we are simply "too young to know better."

Society has long treated lesbians, bisexuals, and gays as though they were errant youths who need help from a proper, "mature" guide. Indeed, for years psychologists claimed that homosexuality was evidence of arrested adolescent development. This outlook justified the punishment and "curing" of homosexuals, who had to be taught to know better. Only in recent times has this attitude "officially" changed. The gay public now asserts its right to be free of this prejudice. But until gay adults do away with their own ageist prejudices and recognize their younger counterparts, gay teens, how can they reasonably expect recognition from the heterosexual public for all bisexuals, lesbians, and gays?

Respect for gay youth must be manifest on a personal basis. A high school student who comes out must be heard. For me, this respect came first from the student who signed himself only "a friend" and responded to my letter to Stephen. Near the end of his letter he wrote, "Just go with what feels right; that's the best advice anyone can tell you," pointing out that I am the only one with insight into my own feelings. Instead of "guidance," what he gave me was affirmation of the identity I'd already formed. Sexuality, he recognized, is not a collaborative effort. Everyone, of every age and every sexuality, must acknowledge the validity of self-definition. As the lesbian faculty member in my dorm said, "If someone is strong enough to be coming out, I know they know what they're talking about" — regardless of their age.

Challenges for Educators: Lesbian, Gay, and Bisexual Families

by James T. Sears

> *Kim and Carolyn, a Boston area lesbian couple, took in Earl, a Black deaf boy, who at the time was five years old. Kim is also deaf, although she can speak and lip-read. . . . Eventually, Kim and Carolyn were formally approved as Earl's foster parents by Massachusetts social workers. Several years later the two women adopted Earl. . . . [At age 11] Earl is a child who is different. He is deaf in a hearing world; Black in a predominantly white community; and the son of [white and Asian] lesbians in a largely heterosexual culture. (Sands 1988, pp. 46-47, 50)*

> *Since I made the decision seven years ago to become a parent through anonymous donor insemination, the question that others have asked most frequently is, "But how are you going to explain this to your child?" . . . During breakfast today, in the middle of a discussion about Velcro closings on shoes, Jonathon [her five-year-old son] asked why he has only a mom and some people have a mom and a dad. I explained that there are all kinds of families in the world and gave lots of examples of those he knows: some with, some without kids; some big, some small. We talked about the fact that from the time I was 15, I just had a dad and no mom.*

---

*This article first appeared in *The High School Journal* 77, nos. 1 and 2 (October-November 1993/December-January 1994), pp. 95-107. Reprinted with permission of the author and the publisher.

I explained that there are no set rules for who family members can be; rather, families are people who love and are there for one another. (Blumenthal 1990/91, p. 45)

The seven-year-old daughter [Alicia] asked her father some questions about "Gene" (the lover), and the father answered them honestly, explaining that he loved Gene and he loved Mommy. The daughter did not seem concerned, but shortly afterward she asked her mother, "Do you still love Daddy?" Mother assured her that she did. "Do you love Gene?" the daughter asked. "He's my friend," her mother answered, "but I love your father." (Matteson 1987, p. 151)

Jennifer sits down at the kitchen table to eat her cereal and juice. "What will you be doing at school, today?" asks Patsy, her mother. "Mrs. Thomkins says we will make Christmas trees today." Patsy's husband, Bill, pours another cup of coffee and says: "Well, I guess that means that we won't have to go and chop down a tree this year!" "Oh, no!" Jennifer exclaims. "We're going to make them out of paper. When are we going to get our tree?" "Well," Patsy's mother says, "When Pam's ship returns for Christmas next week. Until then, you and Bill can talk about where we should go this year for our tree." Jennifer finishes her meal, kisses her mother and Patsy's husband good-bye. "Oh, I almost forgot. Where's Bob?" Bob, Bill's lover of five years, sits in the living room reading the morning paper. "I'm out here, Jennifer. Give me a kiss before you go to school." — An Alabama family (circa 1991)

The traditional American family — to the degree that it ever existed — represents a minority of all households in the United States today (Kamerman and Hayes 1982). There are three major types of American family: families of first marriage, single-parent families, and families of remarriage. Less than one in four students come to school from a home occupied by both biological parents. Single-parent households account for about one-quarter of all American families; about one of every two African-American children (one of every four white children) live with a lone parent (Glick 1988). If current trends continue, six out of ten children will be part of a single family sometime before they become 18 years of age (Bozett and Hanson 1991). These single households are generally the product of divorce or separation. Remarried families account for one in six households, with nearly six million stepchildren (Glick 1987).

In recent years, alternative family arrangements have emerged in which either one or both partners are a self-identified lesbian, gay man, or bisexual person (Alpert 1988; Pollack and Vaughn 1989; Schulenberg 1985).[1] Children, like Jennifer, from these alternative marriages may be the product of a prior marriage in which the partner has custody or visiting privileges or the gay or lesbian couple's decision, like Kim and Carolyn, to adopt (Jullion 1985; Ricketts and Achtenberg 1987).[2] Other children, like Alicia, may live in a biologically traditional family but have one or both parents who are openly bisexual (Matteson 1985; 1987). Children, like Jonathon, may also come to school from households of a lesbian or bisexual woman who has elected to bear and raise the child following artificial insemination or the departure of the father (Pies 1985; 1987). And, of course, the parents of many other children never choose to disclose their bisexuality or homosexuality to their family (Green and Clunis 1989).

The publications on alternative families, such as *Jenny Lives with Eric and Martin* (Bosche 1983), *How Would You Feel if Your Dad Was Gay?* (Heron and Maran 1990), and *Daddy's Roommate* (Wilhoite 1990), as well as the controversy surrounding the New York City Public Schools' adoption of the Rainbow Curriculum and the subsequent dismissal of its superintendent, Frank Fernandez, may mean that few of our students will understand the true diversity among the families whose children attend their schools. Deleting lesbian, gay, and bisexual families from the school curriculum, however, does not remove them from the day-to-day realities of school life. If we are to truly serve all of our students, then educators must become more aware of the challenges facing lesbian, gay, and bisexual parents and their children.

Two of the greatest challenges [for gay and lesbian parents] are securing or maintaining custody of their children and disclosing their homosexuality to their children.

Challenges Facing Lesbian, Gay, and Bisexual Parents

How, the average person wants to know, can a lesbian possibly be a mother? If heterosexual intercourse is the usual prerequisite for maternity, how is it possible for women who by *definition* do not engage in heterosexual behavior to be mothers? If motherhood is a state which requires the expression of nurturance, altruism, and the sacrifice of sex-

189

ual fulfillment, how can a lesbian, a being thought to be oversexed, narcissistic, and pleasure oriented, perform the maternal role? How can women who are "masculine," aggressive, and assumed to be confused about their gender be able to behave appropriately within its boundaries, or to assume the quintessentially womanly task of motherhood? If lesbians are women whose lives are organized in terms of the relentless pursuit of clandestine pleasures, if lesbians are women who behave as quasi-men and who have been poorly socialized into their gender roles, then how can they expect to provide adequate models of feminine behavior to their children, to prepare them for their own sexual and parental careers? (Lewin and Lyons 1982, p. 250)

Such questions pose challenges to women (and men) who are homosexual but choose parenting. While the assumptions underlying many of these questions are flawed (Sears 1991*a*), the coupling of parenthood with homosexuality to form categories of lesbian mothers and gay fathers may appear contradictory. However, this contradiction is of social, not biological, origin.

The difficulties confronted by acknowledged lesbian mothers or gay fathers are, in many ways, similar to those faced by single and divorced parents, with the significant exception of the additional burden of wrestling with the social stigma associated with homosexuality. Two of the greatest challenges are securing or maintaining custody of their children and disclosing their homosexuality to their children.

Legal Barriers. In child custody decisions the judge has a wide leeway within common law to provide for the "best interest of the child" and not to interfere with existing custody arrangements unless there have been "material changes in circumstances" (Achtenburg 1985; Basile 1974; Payne 1977/78). While heterosexual mothers have generally not lost custody of their children for unfitness, the sexual orientation of a parent has played a prominent role in both circumstances (Pagelow 1980; Rivera 1987).

In general, gay fathers seeking custody face the double burden of being male where the female is presumed more nurturant and of being homosexual where heterosexual is considered normal. Moreover, in those cases involving a son, the court appears more concerned with issues of sexual development than in those involving daughters (Miller 1979*b*); and in custody disputes involving lesbian mothers, the woman loses 85% of those cases that go to trial (Chesler 1986). A disproportionate number of cases are between the mother and another relative (Hitchens 1979/80); and in cases where lesbian mothers are provided custody, the courts have often demanded the absence of same-sex lovers in the household. One lesbian who won provisional custody of her five-year-old son lamented:

> That is unjust! They don't put those kinds of restrictions on a heterosexual mother . . . for 13 years I'm forbidden to set up a living relationship with a sexual partner of my choice. Sure, I don't have to be celibate — I can sneak out somewhere or I can send my son away — but I want to be free to set up my home with someone I love. It's much better for a child to have more than one parent figure — I can't possibly be available to answer all of my child's needs alone. (Pagelow 1980, p. 194)

In deciding whether to award custody, or even visiting privileges, to a homosexual parent or to allow a lesbian or gay couple to adopt a child, judges often base their decisions on other unsubstantiated judicial fears, such as "turning" the child into a homosexual, molesting the child, stigmatization of the child, and AIDS (Hitchens 1979/80; Payne 1977/78; Polikoff 1987; Rivera 1987). The willingness of the courts to entertain homosexuality as a factor for denying custody or restricting visiting rights has not escaped the attention of many lesbian mothers who, though themselves not a party to legal action, fear such a possibility (Kirkpatrick, Smith, and Roy 1981).

Non-biological parents and lesbians or gay men wishing to adopt also face significant legal hurdles. Six jurisdictions in the United States have ruled in favor of adoptions by same-sex parents (Alaska, Washington, Oregon, California, Minnesota, and the District of Columbia); and while only two states (Massachusetts and Florida) specifically prohibit gay men or lesbians from being foster or adoptive parents, most courts and agencies have allowed sodomy statutes (applicable in 25 states), prejudicial attitudes, or myths and stereotypes to affect their decisions. In Minnesota, for example, one lesbian was denied visitation rights to a child she had raised with her former partner; and in Wisconsin the court refused to enforce a co-parenting contract signed by two former lovers. Even in states that have ruled in favor of adoptions, there remains bureaucratic and political resistance and, if approved, joint adoptions by gay men or lesbians are unusual (Achtenberg 1985; Ricketts and Achtenberg 1987).

Only recently have education associations, state departments of education, and school districts developed policies and programs regarding the discrimination and harassment of homosexual students or the inclusion of sexual orientation issues in the school curriculum; little attention has been given to children with a lesbian or gay parent. As I will discuss in the final section of this essay, these policies and programs, however, can have a positive affect on not only the lesbian, gay, or bisexual student but also the heterosexual student who comes from such an alternative family structure.

Disclosure to Children. Some, if not most, of our children from such families have not been told of their parent's sexual identity (Bozett 1980; Miller 1979*a*). In heterosexually coupled families with a gay, lesbian, or bisexual spouse, underlying tensions may create home problems (for example, marital discord, emotional detachment from the child) that manifest themselves in a child's school behavior or academic achievement (Harris and Turner 1985/86; Lewis 1980; Matteson 1987). In those families, for example, where gay fathers have not disclosed their sexual identity to their children, Miller (1979*b*) found: "their fathering is of lower quality than the fathering of more overt respondents. . . . The guilt many of these men experienced over being homosexual manifested itself in over-indulgent behavior. . . . Data also indicate that respondents living with their wives tended to spend less time with their children" (p. 550). Educators who are aware of this social phenomenon can integrate this knowledge with their classroom assessment while respecting the confidentiality of the family.

Parents often fear the impact of such disclosure on their children. In deciding whether to disclose the parent's sexual identity, the most common parental fears are rejection from the child, inability of the child to understand, and child rejection from peers (Shernoff 1984; Wyers 1984; 1987). The difficulties faced by the gay or bisexual partner in "coming out" to a child are well articulated by Matteson (1987), following his analysis of a non-clinical sample of 44 spouses in a mixed-orientation marriage:

> *. . . the difficulties of growing up in a lesbian, gay, or bisexual household are linked to the homophobia and heterosexism pervasive in our society and tolerated, if not magnified, in our public schools.*

192

"Since the beginning, I've been saying, 'next year I'm leaving as soon as the children are bigger.' Now that they are in college, I can't leave because they are my judges. They'd never forgive me for doing this all these years to their mother." (p. 145)

The most common time for such disclosure is during a separation or a divorce or when the gay parent elects to enter into a domestic partnership (Bozett 1981b, Miller 1978). In the case of still-married bisexual spouses, somewhere between one-third to one-half of their school-age children have been informed (Coleman 1985; Wolf 1985). The mean age of gay parental self-disclosure or child discovery ranges from 8 to 11 years of age (Turner, Scadden, and Harris 1985; Wyers 1984). According to Bozett (1987b):

> The means by which the father discloses takes several forms. For example, with small children the father may disclose indirectly by taking children to a gay social event or by hugging another man in their presence. Both indirect and direct means may be used with older children in which the father also discusses his homosexuality with them. (p. 13)

Studies of gay parents and their children report different findings regarding the child's reaction (Bozett 1980; Harris and Turner 1985/86; Lewis 1980; Miller 1979b; Paul 1986; Pennington 1987; Turner, Scadden, and Harris 1985; Wyers 1987). In her clinical study of 32 children from 28 lesbian-mother families, Pennington (1987) found the differing "children's reactions to mother 'coming out' generally range from 'Please, can't you change, you're ruining my life!' to 'I'm proud of my mom, and if other kids don't like it, then I don't want that kind of person to be my friend'" (p. 66). In his study of 40 gay fathers, Miller (1979b) on the other hand, found all of their children to have reacted more positively than their fathers had anticipated. Further, "children who showed the greatest acceptance were those who, prior to full disclosure, were gradually introduced by their parents to homosexuality through meeting gay family friends, reading about it, and discussing the topic informally with parents" (p. 549). In general, these and other studies (for example, Gantz 1983; Lamothe 1989; Schulenburg 1985) found the parent-child relationship was ultimately enhanced by such disclosure.

193

Challenges Faced by Children with Lesbian, Gay, or Bisexual Parents

> Susan expected her family to be thrilled that she was finally "settling down" after a decade of working as a lawyer. Her mother's first reaction [to Susan's interest in having a baby], however, was "But you're not married!" After Susan explained that she was still lesbian and planned to raise the child with her lover, Susan's mother wondered, "But is it fair to the child? Everyone else will have a father; she'll feel different, she'll be treated badly." (Rohrbaugh 1989, pp. 51-52)

In the past, concerns about children growing up in a homosexual household focused on the household as the potential problem. Children were believed to be at a higher risk of developing a gender inappropriate identity or sex-typed behaviors, acquiring a homosexual orientation, or exhibiting behavioral or psychological problems. While these fears are unjustified, the difficulties of growing up in a lesbian, gay, or bisexual household are linked to the homophobia and heterosexism pervasive in our society and tolerated, if not magnified, in our public schools.

Impact of Parental Sexual Orientation on Children. As the discussion of gay parenting becomes more public, fears about a child living with a lesbian or gay parent have been expressed. One concern is that the child may become homosexual or experience sexual harassment from either the parent or parental friends. Though persons generally do not identify themselves as gay or lesbian until their late teens or early twenties (Sears 1991*a*; Rust 1993), there is no greater likelihood that a son or daughter of a homosexual parent may declare a homosexual identity than those children from heterosexual households (Bozett 1981*a*; 1981*b*; Gottman 1990; Green 1987; Miller 1979*b*; Paul 1986). Further, there is no empirical evidence that such children living with lesbian or gay parents face any greater danger of sexual harassment or molestation than those living with heterosexual parents (Hotvedt and Mandel 1982; Miller 1979*b*).

Another concern is that children living in homosexual families may suffer in gender development or model "inappropriate" sex-role behaviors. Here research studies present a mixed picture. While some studies have found that homosexual parents, like their heterosexual counterparts, encourage their child's use of sex-typed toys (Golombok, Spencer, and Rutter 1983; Gottman 1990; Harris and Turner 1985/86; Kirkpatrick, Smith, and Roy 1981; McGuire and Alexander 1985; Turner, Scadden, and Harris 1985), others have reported the opposite finding, including a greater emphasis on paternal nurturance or less preference for traditional sex-typed play (Hotvedt and Mandel 1982; Scallen 1981).

In general, studies comparing lesbian or gay men as parents with heterosexual single parents (Bigner and Jacobsen 1989; Kirkpatrick, Smith, and Roy 1981; Lewin and Lyons 1982; Scallen 1981) portray families that are either similar to the heterosexual norm or that excel in socially desirable ways (for example, androgynous parenting behaviors, more child-centered fathers). Though the studies cited in this article varied in their methodology and samples, none found homosexuality to be incompatible with fatherhood or motherhood. Further, these studies do not reveal parenting patterns that would be any less positive than those provided by a heterosexual parent (for example, Bozett 1985; Golombok, Spencer, and Rutter 1983; Hoeffer 1981; Robinson and Skeen 1982).

In fact, those men who are most open about their homosexuality, compared with other homosexual fathers, display fatherhood traits that many professionals consider to be desirable. These fathers, for example, used corporal punishment less often, expressed a strong commitment to provide a nonsexist and egalitarian home environment, and were less authoritarian (Miller 1979b). Similar findings were available for lesbian mothers. For example, in comparing black lesbian with black heterosexual mothers (Hill 1981), the lesbians were found to be more tolerant and treated their male and female children in a more sex equitable manner.

Those fathers and mothers who were the most publicly "out" were most likely to provide a supportive home environment. Ironically, given custody or visiting concerns, as well as the general level of homophobia in society, those parents who are the most candid may be most vulnerable to denial of their parenting rights and visible targets for anti-gay harassment of themselves and their children.

Impact of Homophobia and Heterosexism on Children. The most commonly experienced problem or fear confronting children, most notably adolescents, from lesbian or gay households is rejection or harassment from peers or the fear that others would assume that they, too, are homosexual (Bigner and Bozett 1990; Bozett 1987*a*; Lewis 1980; Paul 1986; Wyers 1987). An anecdote told to Pennington (1987) by a daughter of a lesbian mother illustrates the genuine acceptance of children *prior* to encountering stereotypes and harassment in school:

> When I was around five, my mom and Lois told me they were lesbians. I said good, and thought I want to be just like my mom. Well, when I reached about the fifth grade. . . I heard kids calling someone a faggot as a swear word, and I thought, "My God, they're talking about my mom." (p. 61)

Based on his study of 16 children with a gay or bisexual father, Paul (1986), as well as others (for example, Riddle and Arguelles 1981), found that it was during adolescence that these children had the most difficult time coping with their father's sexuality. An excerpt from a case study, written by a family psychotherapist (Corley 1990) who worked with the two lesbians, Jane and Marge, and their eight children — a family for more than ten years — is illustrative. During the next three years of therapy the family began their first open discussions about the special relationship between the two women and the feelings of their children. The therapist continues:

> Marge's two boys had difficult adjusting to do. . . . By now everyone at their school knew Joe and Tom had two mothers. Both of them had come to their school as the primary parent. The children started to tease them about having "lesbos" for parents. Both of the boys [in their early teens] were rather stout in nature so many fights erupted over the teasing they received. Since Joe and Tom were embarrassed over what the children at school were saying, they usually told the teachers and principal that there was no reason for the fights. When Jane and Marge would question them about the fights, they would equally clam up. . . . Because of the lack of intervention, the boys continued to get in trouble at school and started to act out in other ways. Although the boys were only average students, they always passed. Now they were bringing home failing marks. Since these were the first failing grades for either of them, Jane and Marge felt the situation would improve. Unfortunately, the grade sit-

uation only deteriorated. Several parent conferences were called at school. Although both women showed up at the conferences together, nothing was ever mentioned about the family unit or their relationship. It was not until the family came into therapy that the boys revealed they were having problems. (p. 80)

A prominent researcher in the study of children of gay fathers, Frederick Bozett (1980) relays a similar anecdote from a fourteen-year old boy whose gay father had made several school visits: "All his jewelry was on. The teachers knew he was gay, and all the kids saw him and figured it out. It was obvious. They started calling me names like 'homoson.' It was awful. I couldn't stand it. I hate him for it. I really do" (p. 178).

According to Bozett (1987a), children generally use one of three "social control strategies" to deal with their parent's homosexuality. The first, *boundary control, is* evidenced in the child's control of the parent's behavior, the child's control of their own behavior vis-a-vis their gay parent, and the child's control of others' contact with the parent. Some of these controls are evidenced in an interview with two adolescent girls, both of whom have lesbian parents:

> *Margo*: I try and hide stuff when people walk in, but probably most of my friends know.
>
> *Interviewer:* Do they ever ask you directly?
>
> *Tania:* My friends don't. My mother's girlfriend doesn't live with us. My mom keeps stuff out but I make a point of putting it away when someone is going to come over. . . .
>
> *Margo:* I used to always walk between my mother and Cheryl. I used to make Cheryl walk at the curb and my mother inside and I'd walk right in the middle. . . . So it wouldn't be really obvious. But it probably was. . . . People say, "Why do they live together?" And you make up all these stories and they don't even fit together. . . . My mother tries to make up stories sometimes, but it doesn't work because they make no sense. "Oh my girlfriend, my brother's ex-wife's sister. . . ." I used to be real embarrassed. One of my girlfriends asked me once and I was really embarrassed. I was like, "No! What are you talking about? Where did you get that idea from?" But it turned out that her mother was gay too. (Alpert 1988, pp. 100-102)

Children from some minority families may have a particularly difficult time coping with the homosexuality of a parent . . .

197

The second controlling strategy, *nondisclosure*, is evidenced in the child's refusal to share (and in some cases deny) their parent's homosexuality. One lesbian woman, discussing the difficulties she faced in her daughter's denials, commented:

> When I asked Noelle [now age 13] what she would say if anybody asked her about me she said she would deny it. I was very very hurt. I talked it over with Cathy (a lesbian and a close friend). She said her son . . . had got into a fight at school about her and had come home really upset. . . . She told him that she didn't expect him to fight her battles for her. . . . That was fine by her and that really helped me because I realized I should not expect Noelle to fight my battles either. . . . I actually did tell my children that if they want to deny it that's fine and I think that helped them because they were caught a bit between loyalties. (Lesbian Mothers Group 1989, p. 126).

Some children, however, also employ nondisclosure to protect the parent who might be vulnerable to a child custody challenge or to job discrimination (Paul 1986).

The third controlling strategy, *disclosure*, is evidenced by a child's selective sharing of this personal information. In Miller's (1979*b*) study of gay fathers, one 17-year-old son stated, "I don't tell people if they're uptight types or unless I know them well. I've told my close friends and it's cool with them" (p. 548). In Gantz's (1983) study, a 13-year-old child of a household with two lesbians noted, "I've told one person. . . . We'd go do stuff like shoot pool and all that down in his basement. I just told him, you know, that they were gay. . . . I didn't know how he'd react. He said he'd keep it a secret, so that made me feel a little better" (p. 68). Another male respondent commented, "You have to be sure they won't tell somebody else. I was worried [about] people knowing [because] I was afraid of what they'd think of me; maybe it would be embarrassing" (Bozett 1987*a*, p. 43).

Further, according to Bozett (1987*a*), there are several factors that influence the degree to which children employ one or more of these strategies. Those children who identify with the father because of their behavior, lifestyle, values, or beliefs are less likely to use any social control strategy. Whereas children who view their father's homosexuality as "obtrusive," who are older, or who live with their father are more likely to employ these strategies.

Studies on children from gay families or homosexual mothers and fathers have been conducted within a Euro-American context. Only one study has examined minority homosexual parents (Hill 1981), and there has been no research directed at minority children of a gay parent. Anecdotal writings by persons of color who are homosexual parents, however, convey some dissimilarities with their Anglo counterparts. For example, Lorde (1987) writes:

> Black children of lesbian couples have an advantage because they learn, very early, that oppression comes in many different forms, none of which have anything to do with their own worth. . . . I remember that for years, in the name-calling at school, boys shouted at Jonathan not — "Your mother's a lesbian" — but rather "Your mother's a nigger." (p. 222)

Research into the unique difficulties confronting lesbian or gay young adults who must cope with their emerging homosexual identity within the context of a non-dominant culture underscores the difficulties of being a minority within a minority and suggests differences that minority children with gay or lesbian parents might confront (Johnson 1981; Sears 1991a). Morales (1990) explains:

> What does it mean to be an ethnic minority gay man or lesbian? For ethnic minority gays and lesbians, life is often living in three different communities: the gay/lesbian community, the ethnic minority community, and the predominantly heterosexual white mainstream society. Since these three social groups have norms, expectations, and styles, the minority lesbian or gay man must balance a set of often conflicting challenges and pressures. The multi-minority status makes it difficult for a person to become integrated and assimilated. (p. 220)

This was evident in my study of young lesbian and gay African-American Southerners (Sears 1991a). Irwin, a working-class black man, for example, states: "When you're black in a black society and you're gay it's even harder. Blacks don't want it to be known because they don't want to mimic or im-

199

itate white people. They see it as a crutch and they don't want to have to deal with it" (p. 135). Malcolm comments, "If they are going to see you with a man at all, they would rather see you with another black man. . . . If they think you're gay and you're with a white man, they think that he's your sugar daddy or you're a snow queen" (p.138). This is also evident in the anecdotal and autobiographical writings by people of color (for example, Beam 1986; Moraga and Anzaldua 1981; Smith 1983). A Chinese-American (Lim-Hing 1990/91), for example, writes about her family's reactions to her lesbianism:

> The implicit message my family gave me was not so much a condemnation as an embarrassed tolerance inextricably tied to a plea for secrecy. . . . At the end of my stay [with my father], he asked me if "they" would pick me up at Logan, although he knows Jacquelyn's name. My father's inability to accept my being a lesbian is related to his more traditional values: family first, make money and buy land, don't stand out. (p. 20)

A Puerto Rican (Vazquez 1992) expresses his anger at racism encountered within the Anglo gay community: "I won't lay in my own bed with some Euro-American and do Racism 101. Nor do I want to sit down with the cute white boy I'm dating and deconstruct the statement, 'I love sleeping with Puerto Ricans'" (p. 90).

Children from some minority families may have a particularly difficult time coping with the homosexuality of a parent or may choose to cope with the information in a culturally different manner than researchers such as Bozett have found. Whether it is a child "coming out" to his family, a parent disclosing her homosexual orientation to the children, or both revealing this information to their extended family, they do so within different cultural contexts, perhaps facing greater risks than their Euro-American counterparts. Morales (1990) writes:

> "Coming out" to the family tends to involve both the nuclear and extended family systems. Such a family collective is the major support system for the ethnic persons and is the source of great strength and pride. . . . For minority lesbians and gays coming out to the family not only jeopardizes the intra-family relationships, but also threatens their strong

. . . every major professional educational association has adopted resolutions calling on schools to address this topic [homosexuality].

association with their ethnic community. As a result minority gays and lesbians may run the risk of feeling uprooted as an ethnic person. (p. 233)

Other difficulties faced by both Anglo and minority children of lesbian, gay, and bisexual parents may be the same as those for children from other families experiencing marital discord or integrating a new adult into the household (Hotvedt and Mandel 1982; Miller 1979b; Weeks, Derdeyn, and Langman 1975). Like children of heterosexual divorces, adolescents generally experience the most difficult period of adjustment during the first year of separation. In one of the first studies of gay fathers and their children, Miller (1979b) found "problems of sexual acting out" in the biographies of 48 daughters and 42 sons. Only

> two daughters reported premarital pregnancies and abortions; one admitted to engaging in some prostitution. Two interviewed offspring had problems in school, and one had professional counseling for emotional difficulties. As studies of children of divorced heterosexual parents have revealed similar problems. . . these concerns may not result so much from the father's homosexuality as from family tensions surrounding marital instability, divorce, and residential relocation. Anger and bitterness toward parents are common to children with disrupted families, and respondents in this study were not immune to such feelings. (p. 547)

In another study matching separated or divorced lesbian mothers with heterosexual mothers and using a variety of questionnaires, attitude scales, as well as interviews for both parents and pre-adolescent children (ages 3-11), Hotvedt and Mandel (1982) concluded that there was "no evidence of gender identity conflict, poor peer relationships, or neglect" (p. 285). These findings were extended by Huggins (1989), who examined children's self-esteem through interviews and surveys of 36 adolescents whose head of household was lesbian. Compared with a match-set of heterosexual single female parents, Huggins concluded that "the mother's sexual object choice does not appear to influence negatively the self-esteem of her adolescent children. . . . the assumption that children of lesbian mothers are socially stigmatized by their mothers' sexual choice is not borne out by this study" (p. 132).

While this study does not imply that these children experienced no difficulties because of the stigma of homosexuality, it does mean that "the development of self-esteem is primarily influenced by the interaction between children and their parents or primary caregivers" (Huggins 1989, p.132). For example, one study found that one out of two children of lesbian mothers experienced relationship problems with other people due to the stigma of their mother's sexual identity (Wyers 1987), and another (Lewis 1980) concluded:

> Although the findings are similar to those. . . of children of divorce, the particular issue of acceptance of the "crisis" is dissimilar. . . . Children's initial reaction to divorce was denial of pain; follow-up one year later revealed more open acceptance of the hurt. One reason for this difference may be that children of divorce have community support for their pain; children of lesbians do not. (p. 199)

Of course, parenting by lesbians, gay men, and bisexuals presents society with alternate approaches to family life which can challenge oppressive sexist and heterosexist myths and stereotypes. Sandra Pollack (1989), though acknowledging the legal necessity for demonstrating the sameness between homosexual and heterosexual families, challenges the "underlying assumption that the lesbian mother should be judged on how well she compares to the heterosexual norm." For example, do we really believe that, as a society, we want to foster the continued sex-role education of children?

Pollack argues that rather than accepting the values associated with the heterosexual family, lesbian and gay parenting affords opportunities to challenge these norms in society and in the upbringing of their children. The "possible benefits of being a child of a lesbian mother" include "the children of lesbians may become aware (perhaps more so than other children) of their responsibility for themselves and their choices" (p. 322). For example, one study (Harris and Turner 1985/86) reported that lesbian mothers tended to use their homosexuality in a positive manner through assisting their children to accept their own sexuality, adopt empathetic and tolerant attitudes, and consider other points of view.

Central to the problems faced by children of lesbian and gay parents is the heterosexism and homophobia rampant in today's society. Homophobia — an irrational fear and hatred of homosexuals (Weinberg 1972) — manifests itself in students' negative attitudes and feelings about homosexuality and the institutionalization of sodomy statutes that deny rights of sexual expression among persons of the same gender, thus restricting the legal definition of marriage and family. Heterosexism — the presumption of superiority and exclusiveness of heterosexual relationships — is evidenced in the assumption that parents of all children are heterosexual or that a heterosexual adult will *prima facie* be a better parent than one who is homosexual.

As two leading researchers on gay parenting stated, "Much ignorance regarding homosexuality is due to the propagation of myths. It is important for educators in many disciplines and at all educational levels to dispel myths, impart facts, and promote values clarification" (Bigner and Bozett 1990, p. 168). It is at this juncture that educators' concern for the student with a newly identified lesbian or gay parent is married to their concern for the gay or lesbian student and for the heterosexual student harboring intensely homophobic feelings and attitudes. Each of these students can benefit from honest discussion about homosexuality in the school (Sears 1987; 1991*b*), the adoption and implementation of anti-harassment guidelines (Sears 1992*d*), the portrayal of the contributions and rich history of lesbians, gay men, and bisexuals (Sears 1983), and the provision of gay-affirmative counseling services (Sears 1989*b*).

Based upon her interviews with children with lesbian mothers, Lewis (1980) concurred:

> The children of lesbians seem not to have peer support available to them, since most of these children have either pulled away from their friends altogether or maintained friends but with a sense of their own differentness. Children of lesbians have been taught the same stereotypical myths and prejudices against homosexuals as the rest of society. Better understanding is needed about available family support systems and other systems that should be provided. These might include peer supports as well as educational supports, for example, dissemination of information about homosexuality. (p. 202)

Homosexuality and the Schools

Though some teachers, administrators, and guidance counselors are reluctant to discuss homosexuality in schools (Sears 1992*a*; 1992*b*), every major professional educational association has adopted resolutions calling on schools to address this topic. Some school districts have adopted specific programs and policies, and a variety of recommendations have been made to integrate issues relating to homosexuality in the school curriculum. Educators who assume proactive roles not only benefit lesbian, gay, and bisexual students but are making inroads into the institutionalized homophobia and heterosexism that makes school life more difficult for children from homosexual families.

Gay and Lesbian Students and Professional Standards. Professional education associations have adopted policies affirming the worth and dignity of lesbians, gay men, and bisexuals and/or calling for an end to statutes, policies, and practices that effectively condone discrimination and harassment on the basis of sexual identity. Educators, school board members, and parents who have spearheaded these efforts acknowledge the simple social fact that being sexually different in a society of sexual sameness exacts a heavy psychological toll. Struggling to cope with their sexual identity, these students are more likely than other youth to attempt suicide, to abuse drugs or alcohol, and to experience academic problems (Gibson 1989; Hetrick and Martin 1987; Martin and Hetrick 1988; Sears 1989b; Teague 1992; Zera 1992). Other youth coping with their same-sex feelings may not display these symptoms but may excel in schoolwork, extracurricular activities, or sports as a means of hiding their sexual feelings from themselves or others (Sears 1991a). By hiding, however, their emotional and sexual development languishes (Martin 1982).

Five states (Massachusetts, New Jersey, Wisconsin, Hawaii, and Minnesota) have adopted some type of anti-discrimination statutes. For example, Wisconsin's statute Section 118.13 reads, in part:

> No person may be denied admission to any public school or be denied participation in, be denied the benefits of or be discriminated against in any curricular, extracurricular, pupil services, recreational, or other program or activity because of the person's sex, race... marital or parental status, sexual orientation.

As part of the process of implementing its statute, the Wisconsin Department of Public Instruction issued a 59-page booklet, which noted "the board

204

shall adopt instructional and library media materials selection policies stating that instructional materials, texts, and library services reflect the cultural diversity and pluralist nature of American study" and cited lesbian/gay students as one under-represented group.

Finally, many major education organizations, such as the National Educational Association, American Federation of Teachers, and the Association for Supervision and Curriculum Development, have adopted statements affirming the rights of homosexual/bisexual students in K-12 schools and calling on their members to undertake proactive measures to combat the heterosexism and homophobia that are rampant in our nation's schools. For example, the American School Health Association issued a policy statement on gay and lesbian youth in schools that stated, in part:

> School personnel should discourage any sexually oriented, deprecating, harassing, and prejudicial statements injurious to students' self-esteem. Every school district should provide access to professional counseling by specially trained personnel for students who may be concerned about sexual orientation.

School Polices and Programs. Since the late 1980s, the invisibility of homosexuality in education has lessened. Evidence of its being less invisible includes extensive sex education courses in this nation's schools (Haffner 1990; Sears 1992*c*) with some systems including units on homosexuality (Sears 1991*b*); the first public funding of a school serving homosexual students, The Harvey Milk School, by the New York City public school system (Friends of Project 10 1991; Rofes 1989); the institution of the first gay-affirmative counseling service in a public high school, Project 10 within the Los Angles Unified School District (Rofes 1989); the election of the nation's first openly gay school board member in San Francisco; and the formation of the Lesbian and Gay Studies special interest group of the American Educational Research Association (Grayson 1987).

Several school districts have adopted anti-harassment guidelines. In 1987, the Cambridge (Mass.) public schools included in their policies the following statement:

Harassment on the basis of an individual's sexual preference or orientation is prohibited. Words, action or other verbal, written, or physical conduct which ridicules, scorns, mocks, intimidates, or otherwise threatens an individual because of his/her sexual orientation/preference constitutes homophobic harassment when it has the purpose or effect of unreasonably interfering with the work performance or creating an intimidating, hostile, or offensive environment. (Peterkin 1987)

More recently, in 1991, the St. Paul school board passed a human rights policy forbidding discrimination on the basis of "sexual or affectional orientation." Several large urban school districts (for example, New York, Washington, D.C., Cincinnati, Los Angeles, Des Moines, San Francisco) have implemented anti-gay and lesbian discrimination policies. Perhaps the most publicized effort to meet the needs of homosexual students has been the funding of a public alternative school for gay and lesbian youth in New York City and the development of counseling services expressly for this target population in Los Angeles. The Harvey Milk School, established in 1985 under the sponsorship of the Hetrick-Martin Institute, serves about 40 students who are unable to function in the conventional school setting (Rofes 1989). In Los Angeles, Project 10 at Fairfax High School has received international attention for the gay-affirmative services provided by its counseling staff. And, in 1993, the school district, under the auspices of Project 10, hosted the first conference for their high school gay youth at nearby Occidental College.

These policies and programs not only have a positive impact on the gay, lesbian, and bisexual student but on heterosexual students, faculty, and staff who often harbor homophobic feelings or heterosexist attitudes. Thus, these policies and programs can help to create a supportive school climate for heterosexual students who come from lesbian, gay, or bisexual households.

Curriculum and Staffing Recommendations. Elsewhere (Sears 1987; 1991*b;* 1992*b*) I have discussed the importance of integrating issues of homosexuality into the school curriculum. Briefly, when the issue of homosexuality appears in the school curriculum the most likely subjects to be targeted are science in the form of human physiology or health in the form of HIV/AIDS prevention (Sears 1992*c*). In contrast, I believe, sexuality can serve as a transformative tool for thinking about the construction of one's sexual identities vis-a-vis the interrelationships among language, history, and society (Carlson 1992; Macanghaill 1991). As such, sexuality no longer becomes the province of sex educators teaching separate units within physical education or biology but becomes a major strand woven throughout the curriculum (Sears 1991*b*).

Educators have long argued that schools ought to be an embryonic environment for engaging young people in the art of democratic living and, in the process, moving society further along its democratic path (Dewey 1916; Giroux 1988; Rugg 1939). In fact, however, the hidden curriculum of school fosters conformity and passivity while seldom encouraging critical thinking, ethical behavior, and civic courage (Giroux 1988; McLaren 1991; 1993). Within this environment, controversial ideas and individual differences are seldom welcomed. The discussion of homosexuality, the treatment of lesbian, gay, and bisexual students, and the restrictive definition of family are some of the most glaring examples.

Specific strategies and materials that foster an awareness of homosexuality and homosexual persons already have been proposed or developed (for example, Friends of Project 10 1991; Goodman 1983; Hubbard 1989; Krysiak 1987; Lipkin 1992; Sears 1983; Wilson 1984). Educators have been admonished by scholars and activists alike to sit down and talk with bisexual, lesbian, and gay adults to learn firsthand about the special problems they faced in school; the importance of lesbian and gay educators as role models for homosexual students has been stressed, as has the need for public school systems to follow the lead of communities such as Berkeley and Cambridge in adopting anti-slur policies and non-harassment guidelines (Griffin 1992; Hetrick and Martin 1987; Kissen 1991; Martin and Hetrick 1988; Peterkin 1987; Rofes 1989; Sears 1987; 1993; Slater 1988; Stover 1992). In some schools, anti-homophobia workshops with heterosexual students and educators have been conducted (Schneider and Tremble 1986; Stewart 1984). Professional educators as well as lesbian and gay activists ask, at the very least, for the construction of a nonjudgemental atmosphere in which homosexual-identified students can come to terms with their sexuality, the acquisition by school libraries of biographical books where students can discover the homosexuality of some famous people, and the integration of references to homosexual men and women as well as the topic of homosexuality into the high school curriculum (Jenkins 1990; Sears 1983; 1988).

It should be noted that there is no legal justification for systematically barring discussion of homosexuality and the inclusion of the contributions of lesbian, gay, and bisexual artists, politicians, scientists, and athletes from the school curriculum. A United States Court of Appeals ruling that a state statute prohibiting educators and school staff from "advocating, soliciting, or promoting homosexual activity" was unconstitutional was let stand due to a deadlock Supreme Court vote *(National Gay Task Force* v. *Board of Education of the City of Oklahoma,* 1984). Nevertheless, the integration of lesbian, gay, and bisexual topics or persons in the school curriculum appears too radical for many educators. Too few administrators refuse to acquiesce to a scissors-and-paste mentality of curriculum development in which only the most mundane, least controversial material survives the scrutiny of self-appointed moral vigilantes or the self-censorship of timid school officials (Sears 1992*d*; Summerford 1987; Tabbert 1988).

In such an Orwellian school world, the curriculum is carefully crafted to omit (without the appearance of omission) the homoerotic imagery in the poetry of Walt Whitman, Sappho, and Langston Hughes or the visual arts of Donatello, Marsden Hartley, and Robert Mapplethorpe; the conflict between racial and sexual identities present in the literature of James Baldwin, Yukio Mishima, and Toni Morrison; or the conflict between the professional and personal lives of computer inventor Alan Turing, sports heroes David Kopay and Martina Navratilova, and political activists Eleanor Roosevelt and Susan B. Anthony. Just as sexuality is extracted from life and compartmentalized into units of sexuality education, so, too, is bisexuality and homosexuality exorcised from the body politic and tucked away in the curriculum closet.

In each of these areas, educators can play an important role in reducing homophobia and heterosexism. In the process, they can directly counter those litigants who petition courts to deny custody or visitation rights to lesbian or gay parents due to the fear of a "definite possibility of peer ridicule in the future" (Hitchens 1979/80, p. 90).

Summary of Research

Studies on bisexual and homosexual parenting as well as children of lesbians and gay men are far from complete. There are, however, some suggestive findings:

- Children are less accepting when a same-sex parent "comes out" than when a parent of the other gender discloses sexual identity.
- Children of a lesbian or gay parent are no more likely to define themselves as homosexual than children of heterosexual parents, nor are they any more likely to display atypical sex role preferences.
- Lesbian, gay, and bisexual parents often seek to provide children with a variety of gender role models.
- The earlier the disclosure to the child, the fewer problems in the parent/child relationship.
- Children of a lesbian or gay parent follow typical developmental patterns of acquiring sex role concepts and sex-typed behaviors.
- Children of homosexual parents who have experienced marital turmoil face similar difficulties common to children of divorce.
- Gay fathers may have a more difficult time disclosing their sexuality to their children than lesbian mothers, children of gay fathers are less likely to know of their parents sexual identity, and the coming out process is more difficult for gay fathers with children at home.
- Sons are less accepting when learning their parent is gay than are daughters.
- As children enter adolescence, there is a greater likelihood that they will experience peer harassment about their parents' sexual identity and engage in a variety of self-protective mechanisms.
- Gay fathers are more likely to report their children experiencing difficulty with peer harassment because of the parent's homosexuality.

Recommendations for Educators

In several studies, researchers have noted the important role that educators can play in reducing homophobia and heterosexism that create difficult environments for children of lesbian or gay families to learn and for their parents to visit. Based upon these and other writings (for example, Casper and Wickens 1992; Clay 1990), educators should:

- Redesign school paperwork in order to be inclusive. Replace such words as "mother" and "father" with "parent" or "parent 1, parent 2."
- When establishing associations such as parent-teacher organizations, develop assistance for single-parent families (for example, child care) and

create or identify a safe space for homosexual parents (for example, support groups). Encouraging gay parents to share with school officials' their family status is important. Based on his extensive research with children of gay fathers, Bozett (1987a) states:

> It is best for school officials to know about the father's homosexuality, especially if the father has child custody. Knowing about the family can alert school personal to problems which may have the home situation as their genesis. Likewise, if the father is known about by school officials, both the father and his lover may participate in school affairs, attend school functions, or the lover may pick the child up at school all without the parents or the child having to make elaborate explanations. (p. 53)

- Represent family/cultural diversity in classroom materials and books, on bulletin boards, and in everyday teaching practices.
- Insure that books depicting alternative family patterns are included in school libraries (see following resource section for a few recommendations).
- Sensitize teachers and prepare guidance counselors to work with children as well as their gay parent as they confront issues ranging from the child's need for self-protection to the parent's need of respect for their sexual choices.
- Provide role models of gay or lesbian parents for students. Examples should reflect a multicultural emphasis rather than reinforcing the stereotype of homosexuality existing only within the white community. Since some children in every school will identify themselves as lesbian or gay, it is important for them to have positive parenting role models, should they elect to bear or foster children as adults.
- Inform parents of any sexual harassment or intimidation directed at their child.
- Modify the school's anti-slur and anti-harassment policy to include sexual orientation and equally enforce violations against this policy.
- Interview potential teachers and counselors to ascertain their professional experiences and personal attitudes in working with sexual minorities.
- Revise hiring policies and procedures to enhance the likelihood of recruiting sexual minority faculty.

- Develop and publicize a counseling service for students who wish to discuss issues related to sexual identity.
- Hold a series of informal faculty meetings with gay and lesbian parents and faculty to identify needs and possible solutions.
- Meet with support services personnel (for example, media specialists, counselors) to determine the adequacy of resource materials available for students and faculty about homosexuality and bisexuality.
- Review and revise accordingly student and faculty school-sanctioned activities that discriminate on the basis of sexual orientation (for example, Junior ROTC, school dances, job recruitment fairs).
- Review school textbooks for biased or misleading information about lesbians, gays, and bisexuals.
- Review the school curriculum to identify areas within *every* subject where relevant information (people, places, events) about lesbians, gay men, and bisexuals can be included.
- Engage teachers and administrators in formal activities that address the cognitive, affective, and behavioral dimensions of homophobia.
- Develop prejudice awareness among student leaders through after-school workshops.
- Invite former students and members of the community to address the student body on issues relating to homosexuality.

Resources for Educators

There is a wide selection of books, as well as organizations and journals, appropriate for adults interested in lesbian and gay parents or their children. These include:

Alpert, H. *We Are Everywhere: Writings By and About Lesbian Parents.* Freedom, Calif.: Crossing Press, 1988.

Boys of Lesbian Mothers. 935 W. Broadway, Eugene, OR 97402.

Chain of Life. A newsletter for lesbian and gay adoptees. Box 8081, Berkeley, CA 94707.

Children of Gay/Lesbians. 8306 Wilshire Blvd., Suite 222, Beverly Hills, CA 90211.

Empathy: An Interdisciplinary Journal for Persons Working to End Oppression Based on Sexual Identities. Published twice a year (individuals $15, institutions $20), this 100+ page journal regularly includes essays on alternative family structures and issues relating to lesbian, gay, and bisexual youth. PO Box 5085, Columbia, SC 29250.

Gay and Lesbian Parents Coalition International. An advocacy/support group for lesbian and gay parents with a quarterly newsletter. PO Box 50360, Washington, DC 20091.

Gay Fathers. *Some of Their Stories, Experience, and Advice*. Toronto, 1981.

Gay Fathers Coalition. Box 50360, Washington, DC 20004.

Gay Parents Support Packet. National Gay Task Force, 80 Fifth Ave., Room 506, New York, NY 10011.

Jenkins, C. "Being Gay: Gay/Lesbian Characters and Concerns in Young Adult Books." *Booklist*, 1 September 1990, pp. 39-41.

Jullion, J. *Long Way Home: The Odyssey of a Lesbian Mother and Her Children*. Pittsburgh, Pa.: Cleis, 1985.

MacPike, L. *There's Something I've Been Meaning to Tell You*. Tallahassee: Naiad Press, 1989.

Parents and Friends of Lesbians and Gays. PO Box 27605, Washington, DC 20038-7605.

Pollack, S., and Vaughn, J., ed. *Politics of the Heart: A Lesbian Parenting Anthology*. Ithaca, N.Y.: Firebrand, 1989.

Rafkin, L. *Different Mothers: Sons and Daughters of Lesbians Talk About Their Lives*. Pittsburgh, Pa.: Cleis, 1990.

Schulenburg, J. *Gay Parenting: A Complete Guide for Gay Men and Lesbians with Children*. Garden City, N.Y.: Anchor, 1985.

Wolf, V. "The Gay Family in Literature for Young People." *Children's Literature in Education* 20, no. 1 (1989): 51-58.

Footnotes

1. These real-world vignettes reflect the variety of lesbian, gay, or bisexual families. While the number of children of lesbian, gay, and bisexual parents is speculative, researchers cite a range of 6 million to 14 million children (Bozett 1987*a*; Rivera 1987; Schulenberg 1985). Empirical data, itself subject to sampling problems, suggests that approximately one in five lesbians and one in ten gay men have children (Bell and Weinberg 1978; Jay

and Young 1979) with estimates of upwards of 1.5 million lesbians living with their children (Hoeffer 1981). Until recently, these children were the result of defunct heterosexual relationships or marriages in which a spouse's homosexuality remains undisclosed (Brown 1976; Green 1987; Miller 1979*a*).

Studies on lesbian and gay parents and their families have been limited in terms of sample size and methodology. For example, some studies (for example, Weeks, Derdeyn, and Langman 1975) have been clinical case studies and others have relied on anecdotal evidence (for example, Alpert 1988; Brown 1976; Mager 1975); others have studied small (10-40) groups of homosexual parents identified through gay-related organizations (for example, Scallen 1981). Only a few studies have used larger samples with more sophisticated research designs (for example, Bigner and Jacobsen 1989; Hotvedt and Mandel 1982). There have been no ethnographic, longitudinal, or nationwide studies conducted. Further, researchers generally have compared homosexual single parents with single heterosexual parents and, occasionally, homosexual parents living with a domestic partner with remarried heterosexual couples. Due to their incompatibility, no comparisons between homosexual-parented households with the "traditional" two-parent heterosexual families have been made. Further, few of these studies present statistical analyses, control for the presence of a male role model in the home, take into account the desire to appear socially acceptable, include a majority of adolescent subjects, or focus on bisexual parents (Gottman 1990). Finally, only a handful of studies have directly interviewed, surveyed, or observed children raised by a father or mother who is homosexual (Bozett 1980; 1987*b*; Green 1987; Huggins 1989; Paul 1986). For a review of much of this literature, see Bozett (1989).

2. One tragedy of failures to successfully challenge state sodomy statutes in the courts and the legislature is the difficulty that lesbians, gay men, or bisexuals have in obtaining child custody or visiting privileges in divorce hearings or approval from adoption agencies even for children whose prospects for adoption are slim, such as an older child or an HIV-infected baby (Hitchens 1979/80; Payne 1977/78; Ricketts and Achtenberg 1987; Rivera 1987).

References

Achtenburg, R. *Sexual Orientation and the Law*. New York: Clark-Boardman, 1985.

Alpert, H. *We Are Everywhere: Writings By and About Lesbian Parents*. Freedom, Calif.: Crossing Press, 1988.

Basile, R. "Lesbian Mothers and Custody and Homosexual Parents." *Women's Rights Law Reporter* 2 (1974): 3-25.

Beam, J., ed. *In the Life: A Black Gay Anthology*. Boston: Alyson, 1986.

Bell, A., and Weinberg, M. *Homosexualities*. New York: Simon and Schuster, 1978.

Bigner, J., and Bozett, F. "Parenting by Gay Fathers." In *Homosexuality and Family Relations*, edited by F. Bozett and M. Sussman. New York: Haworth Press, 1990.

Bigner, J., and Jacobsen, R. "Parenting Behaviors of Homosexual and Heterosexual Fathers." In *Homosexuality and the Family*, edited by F. Bozett. New York: Haworth Press, 1989.

Blumenthal. A. "Scrambled Eggs and Seed Daddies: Conversations with my Son." *Empathy* 2, no. 2 (1990/1991): 45-48.

Bosche, S. *Jenny Lives with Eric and Martin*. London: Gay Men's Press, 1983.

Bozett, F. "Gay Fathers: How and Why Gay Fathers Disclose Their Homosexuality to Their Children." *Family Relations* 29 (1980): 173-79.

Bozett, F. "Gay Fathers: Evolution of the Gay Father Identity." *American Journal of Orthopsychiatry* 51 (1981): 552-59. a

Bozett, F. "Gay Fathers: Identity Conflict Resolution Through Integrative Sanctions." *Alternative Lifestyles* 4 (1981): 90-107. b

Bozett, F. "Gay Men as Fathers." In *Dimensions of Fatherhood*, edited by S. Hanson and F. Bozett. Beverly Hills, Calif.: Sage, 1985.

Bozett, F. "Children of Gay Fathers." In *Gay and Lesbian Parents*, edited by F. Bozett. Westport, Conn.: Praeger, 1987. a

Bozett, F. "Gay Fathers." In *Gay and Lesbian Parents*, edited by F. Bozett. Westport, Conn.: Praeger, 1987. b

Bozett, F. "Gay Fathers: A Review of the Literature. " In *Homosexuality and the Family*, edited by F. Bozett. New York: Haworth Press, 1989.

Bozett, F., and Hanson, S. "Cultural Change and the Future of Fatherhood and Families." In *Fatherhood and Families in Cultural Context*, edited by F. Bozett and S. Hanson. New York: Springer, 1991.

Brown, H. "Married Homosexuals." In *Familiar Faces, Hidden Lives*, edited by H. Brown. New York: Harcourt Brace Jovanovich, 1976.

Carlson, D. "Ideological Conflict and Change in the Sexuality Curriculum." In *Sexuality and the Curriculum*, edited by J. Sears. New York: Teachers College Press, 1992.

Casper, V., and Wickens, E. "Gay and Lesbian Parents: Their Children in School." *Teachers College Record* 94, no. 1 (1992).

Chesler, P. *Mothers on Trial: The Battle for Children and Custody*. New York: McGraw-Hill, 1986.

Clay, J. "Working with Lesbian and Gay Parents and Their Children." *Young Children* 45, no. 3 (1990): 31-35.

Coleman, E. "Bisexual Women in Marriages." *Journal of Homosexuality* 11 (1985): 87-100.

Corley, R. *The Final Closet*. North Miami, Fla.: Editech Press, 1990.

Dewey, J. *Democracy and Education: An Introduction to the Philosophy of Education*. New York: Macmillan, 1916.

Friends of Project 10. *Project 10 Handbook: Addressing Lesbian and Gay Issues in Our Schools.* 3rd ed. Los Angeles, 1991. ERIC Reproduction No. ED 337 567.

Gantz, J. "The Weston/Roberts Family." In *Whose Child Cries: Children of Gay Parents Talk About Their Lives*, edited by J. Gantz. Rolling Hills Estate, Calif.: Jalmar Press, 1983.

Gibson, P. "Gay Male and Lesbian Youth Suicide." In *Report of the Secretary's Task Force on Youth Suicide. Volume 3: Prevention and Interventions in Youth Suicide.* Washington, D.C.: U.S. Department of Health and Human Services, 1989.

Giroux, H. *Teachers as Intellectuals: Toward a Critical Pedagogy of Learning.* Boston: Bergin & Garvey, 1988.

Glick, P. "Remarried Families, Stepfamilies and Stepchildren." Paper presented at the Wingspread Conference on the Remarried Family. Racine, Wisconsin, 1987.

Glick, P. "Fifty Years of Family Demography: A Record of Social Change." *Journal of Marriage and the Family* 50, no. 4 (1988): 861-73.

Golombok. S.; Spencer, A.; and Rutter, M. "Children in Lesbian and Single-Parent Households: Psychosexual and Psychiatric Appraisal." *Journal of Child Psychology and Psychiatry* 24 (1983): 551-72.

Goodman, J. "Out of the Closet by Paying the Price." *Interracial Books for Children* 9, no. 314 (1983): 13-15.

Gottman, J. "Children of Gay and Lesbian Parents." In *Homosexuality and Family Relations*, edited by F. Bozett and M. Sussman. New York: Haworth Press, 1990.

Grayson, D. "Emerging Equity Issues Related to Homosexuality in Education." *Peabody Journal of Education* 64, no. 4 (1987): 132-45.

Green, G. "Lesbian Mothers." Paper presented at the Annual Convention of the American Psychological Association, 28 August 1987. ERIC Reproduction No. ED 297 205.

Green, G., and Clunis, D. "Married Lesbians." In *Lesbianism: Affirming Nontraditional Roles*, edited by E. Rothblum and E. Cole. New York: Haworth Press, 1989.

Green, R. "Sexual Identity of 37 Children Raised by Homosexual or Transsexual Parents." *American Journal of Psychiatry* 135, no. 6 (1978): 692-97.

Griffin, P. "From Hiding Out to Coming Out: Empowering Lesbian and Gay Educators." In *Homosexuality and Education*, edited by K. Harbeck. New York: Haworth Press, 1992.

Haffner, D. *Sex Education 2000: A Call to Action.* New York: SIECUS, 1990.

Harris, M., and Turner, P. "Gay and Lesbian Parents." *Journal of Homosexuality* 12, no. 2 (1985/1986): 101-13.

Heron, A., and Maran, M. *How Would You Feel if Your Dad Was Gay?* Boston: Alyson, 1990.

Hetrick, E., and Martin, A.D. "Developmental Issues and Their Resolution for Gay and Lesbian Adolescents." *Journal of Homosexuality* 14, nos. 1-2 (1987): 25-43.

Hill, M. "Effects of Conscious and Unconscious Factors on Child Reacting Attitudes of Lesbian Mothers." Doctoral dissertation, Adelphia University, 1981. Dissertation Abstracts International, 42, 1608B.

Hitchens, D. "Social Attitudes, Legal Standards, and Personal Trauma in Child Custody Cases." *Journal of Homosexuality* 5, nos. 1 and 2 (1979/1980): 89-95.

Hoeffer, B. "Children's Acquisition of Sex Role Behavior in Lesbian-Mother Families." *American Journal of Orthopsychiatry* 51, no. 31 (1981): 536-544.

Hotvedt, M., and Mandel, J. "Children of Lesbian Mothers." In *Homosexuality: Social, Psychological, and Biological Issues*, edited by W. Paul, J. Weinrich, J. Gonsiorek, and M. Hotvedt. Beverly Hills, Calif.: Sage, 1982.

Hubbard, B. *Entering Adulthood: Living in Relationships. A Curriculum for Grades 9-12*. Santa Cruz, Calif.: Network Publications, 1989.

Huggins, S. "A Comparative Study of Self-Esteem of Adolescent Children of Divorced Lesbian Mothers and Divorced Heterosexual Mothers." In *Homosexuality and the Family*, edited by F. Bozett. New York: Haworth Press, 1989.

Jay, K., and Young, A. *The Gay Report*. New York: Summit, 1979.

Jenkins, C. "Being Gay: Gay/Lesbian Characters and Concerns in Young Adult Books." *Booklist*, 1 September 1990, pp. 39-41.

Johnson. J. "Influence of Assimilation on the Psychosocial Adjustment of Black Homosexual Men." Doctoral dissertation, California School of Professional Psychology, Berkeley, 1981. Dissertation Abstracts International 42, 11, 4620B.

Jullion, J. *Long Way Home: The Odyssey of a Lesbian Mother and Her Children*. Pittsburgh, Pa.: Cleis, 1985.

Kamerman, S., and Hayes, C. "Families that Work." In *Children in a Changing World*, edited by S. Kamerman and C. Hayes. Washington, D.C.: National Academy Press, 1982.

Kirkpatrick, M.; Smith, C.; and Roy, R. "Lesbian Mothers and Their Children: A Comparative Study." *American Journal of Orthopsychiatry* 51, no. 3 (1981): 545-51.

Kissen, R. "Listening to Gay and Lesbian Teenagers." Paper presented at the Annual Meeting of the National Council of Teachers of English, Seattle, 1991. ERIC Reproduction No. ED 344 220.

Krysiak, G. "Very Silent and Gay Minority." *School Counselor* 34, no. 4 (1987): 304-307.

Lamothe, D. "Previously Heterosexual Lesbian Mothers Who Have Come Out to an Adolescent Daughter: An Exploratory Study of the Coming Out Process." Doctoral dissertation, Antioch University, 1989. Dissertation Abstracts International 50, 5, 2157B.

Lesbian Mothers Group. "A Word Might Slip and that Would Be It." In *Girls and Sexuality: Teaching and Learning*, edited by L. Holly. Milton Keynes: Open University, 1989.

Lewin, E., and Lyons, T. "Everything in Its Place: The Coexistence of Lesbianism and Motherhood." In *Homosexuality: Social, Psychological, and Biological Issues*, edited by W. Paul, J. Weinrich, J. Gonsiorek, and M. Hotvedt. Beverly Hills, Calif.: Sage, 1982.

Lewis, K. "Children of Lesbians: Their Points of View." *Social Work* 25, no. 3 (1980): 198-203.

Lim-Hing, S. "Dragon Ladies, Snow Queens, and Asian-American Dykes: Reflections on Race and Sexuality." *Empathy* 2, no. 2 (1990/1991): 20-22.

Lipkin, A. "Project 10: Gay and Lesbian Students Find Acceptance in Their School Community." *Teaching Tolerance* 1, no. 2 (1992): 24-27.

Lorde, A. "Man Child: A Black Lesbian Feminist's Response." In *Politics of the Heart: A Lesbian Parenting Anthology*, edited by S. Pollack and J. Vaughn. Ithaca, N.Y.: Firebrand, 1987.

Macanghaill, M. "Schooling, Sexuality and Male Power: Towards an Emancipator Curriculum." *Gender and Education* 3, no. 3 (1991): 291-309.

Mager, D. "Faggot Father." In *After You're Out*, edited by K. Jay and A. Young. New York: Gage, 1975.

Martin, A.D. "Learning to Hide: The Socialization of the Gay Adolescent." In *Adolescent Psychiatry: Developmental and Clinical Studies*, edited by S. Feinstein and J. Looney. Chicago: University of Chicago Press, 1982.

Martin, A.D., and Hetrick, E. "The Stigmatization of Gay and Lesbian Adolescents." *Journal of Homosexuality* 15, nos. 1-2 (1988): 163-85.

Matteson, D. "Bisexual Men in Marriages: Is a Positive Homosexual Identity and Stable Marriage Possible?" *Journal of Homosexuality* 11 (1985): 149-73.

Matteson, D. "The Heterosexually Married Gay and Lesbian Parent." In *Gay and Lesbian Parents*, edited by F. Bozett. Westport, Conn.: Praeger, 1987.

McGuire, M., and Alexander, N. "Artificial Insemination of Single Women." *Fertility and Sterility* 43 (1985): 182-84.

McLaren, P. "Critical Pedagogy: Constructing an Arch of Social Dreaming and a Doorway to Hope." *Journal of Education* 173, no. 1 (1991): 9-34.

McLaren, P. *Schooling as a Ritual Performance*. 2nd ed. London: Routledge, 1993.

Miller, B. "Adult Sexual Resocialization: Adjustments Toward a Stigmatized Identity." *Alternative Lifestyles* 1 (1978): 207-34.

Miller, B. "Unpromised Paternity: The Lifestyles of Gay Fathers." In *Gay Men: The Sociology of Male Homosexuality*, edited by M. Levin. New York: Harper & Row, 1979. a

Miller, B. "Gay Fathers and Their Children." *Family Coordinator* 28, no. 4 (1979): 544-52. b

Moraga, C., and Anzaldua, G., ed. *This Bridge Called My Back: Writings by Radical Women of Color*. Watertown, Mass.: Persephone Press, 1981.

Morales, E. "Ethnic Minority Families and Minority Gays and Lesbians." In *Homosexuality and Family Relations*, edited by F. Bozett and M. Sussman. New York: Haworth Press, 1990.

National Gay Task Force v. Board of Education of the City of Oklahoma, State of Oklahoma, 729 Fed.2d 1270 (1984), 33 FEP 1009 (1982).

Pagelow, M. "Heterosexual and Lesbian Single Mothers: A Comparison of Problems, Coping, and Solutions." *Journal of Homosexuality* 5, no. 3 (1980): 189-204.

Paul, J. "Growing Up with a Gay, Lesbian or Bisexual Parent: An Exploratory Study of Experiences and Perceptions." Doctoral dissertation, University of California-Berkeley, 1986. Dissertation Abstracts International, 47, 7, 2756A.

Payne, A. "Law and the Problem Patient: Custody and Parental Rights of Homosexual, Mentally Retarded, Mentally Ill, and Incarcerated Patients." *Journal of Family Law* 16, no. 4 (1977/1978): 797-818.

Pennington, S. "Children of Lesbian Mothers." In *Gay and Lesbian Parents*, edited by F. Bozett. Westport, Conn.: Praeger, 1987.

Peterkin, R. "Letter to Administrative Staff: Anti-Harassment Guidelines." Cambridge, Mass., 11 June 1987

Pies, C. *Considering Parenthood*. San Francisco: Spinster's Ink, 1985.

Pies, C. "Considering Parenthood: Psychosocial Issues for Gay Men and Lesbians Choosing Alternative Fertilization." In *Gay and Lesbian Parents*, edited by F. Bozett. Westport, Conn.: Praeger, 1987.

Polikoff, N. "Lesbian Mothers, Lesbian Families: Legal Obstacles, Legal Challenges." In *Politics of the Heart: A Lesbian Parenting Anthology*, edited by S. Pollack and J. Vaughn. Ithaca, N.Y.: Firebrand, 1987.

Pollack, S. "Lesbian Mothers: A Lesbian-Feminist Perspective on Research." In *Politics of the Heart: A Lesbian Parenting Anthology*, edited by S. Pollack and J. Vaughn. Ithaca, N.Y.: Firebrand, 1989.

Pollack, S., and Vaughn, J., ed. *Politics of the Heart: A Lesbian Parenting Anthology*. Ithaca, N.Y.: Firebrand, 1989.

Ricketts, W., and Achtenberg, R. "The Adoptive and Foster Gay and Lesbian Parent." In *Gay and Lesbian Parents*, edited by F. Bozett. Westport, Conn.: Praeger, 1987.

Riddle, D., and Arguelles, M. "Children of Gay Parents: Homophobia's Victims." In *Children of Separation and Divorce*, edited by I. Stuart and L. Abt. New York: Von Nostrand Reinhold, 1981.

Rivera, K. "Legal Issues in Gay and Lesbian Parenting." In *Gay and Lesbian Parents*, edited by F. Bozett. Westport, Conn.: Praeger, 1987.

Robinson, B., and Skeen, P. "Sex-Role Orientation of Gay Fathers Versus Gay Nonfathers." *Perceptual and Motor Skills* 55 (1982): 1055-1059.

Rofes, E. "Opening Up the Classroom Closet: Responding to the Educational Needs of Gay and Lesbian Youth." *Harvard Educational Review* 59, no. 4 (1989): 444-53.

Rohrbaugh, J. "Choosing Children: Psychological Issues in Lesbian Parenting." In *Lesbianism: Affirming Nontraditional Roles*, edited by E. Rothblum and E. Cole. New York: Haworth Press, 1989.

Rugg, H. *Democracy and the Curriculum: The Life and Progress of the American School*. New York: Appleton-Century, 1939.

Rust, P. "'Coming Out' in the Age of Social Constructions: Sexual Identity Formation Among Lesbian and Bisexual Women." *Gender and Society* 7, no. 1 (1993): 50-77.

Sands, A. "We Are Family." In *We Are Everywhere: Writings By and About Lesbian Parents*, edited by H. Alpert. Freedom, Calif.: Crossing Press, 1988.

Scallen, R. "An Investigation of Paternal Attitudes and Behaviors in Homosexual and Heterosexual Fathers." Doctoral dissertation, California School of Professional Psychology, Los Angeles, 1981. Dissertation Abstracts International, 42, 9, 3809B.

Schneider, M., and Tremble, B. "Training Service Providers to Work with Gay or Lesbian Adolescents: A Workshop." *Journal of Counseling and Development* 65, no. 2 (1986): 98-99.

Schulenberg, J. *Gay Parenting*. New York: Doubleday, 1985.

Sears, J. "Sexuality: Taking Off the Masks." *Changing Schools* 11 (1983): 12-13.

Sears, J. "Peering into the Well of Loneliness: The Responsibility of Educators to Gay and Lesbian Youth." In *Social Issues and Education: Challenge and Responsibility*, edited by Alex Molar. Alexandria, Va.: Association for Supervision and Curriculum Development, 1987.

Sears, J. "Growing Up Gay: Is Anyone There to Listen?" *American School Counselors Association Newsletter* 26 (1988): 8-9.

Sears, J. "The Impact of Gender and Race on Growing Up Lesbian and Gay in the South." *NASA Journal* 1, no. 3 (1989): 422-57. a

Sears, J. "Counseling Sexual Minorities: An Interview with Virginia Uribe." *Empathy* 1, no. 2 (1989): 1, 8. b

Sears, J. *Growing Up Gay in the South: Race, Gender, and Journeys of the Spirit*. New York: Haworth Press, 1991. a

Sears, J. "Teaching for Diversity: Student Sexual Identities." *Educational Leadership* 49 (1991): 54-57. b

Sears, J. "Educators, Homosexuality, and Homosexual Students: Are Personal Feelings Related to Professional Beliefs?" *Journal of Homosexuality* (1992): 29-79. a

Sears, J. "The Impact of Culture and Ideology on the Construction of Gender and Sexual Identities: Developing a Critically-Based Sexuality Curriculum." In *Sexuality and the Curriculum: The Politics and Practices of Sexuality Education*, edited by J. Sears. New York: Teachers College Press, 1992. b

Sears, J. "Dilemmas and Possibilities of Sexuality Education: Reproducing the Body Politic." In *Sexuality and the Curriculum: The Politics and Practices of Sexuality Education*, edited by J. Sears. New York: Teachers College Press, 1992. c

Sears, J. "Responding to the Sexual Diversity of Faculty and Students: An Agenda for Critically Reflective Administrators." In *The Social Context of Education: Administration in a Pluralist Society*, edited by C. Capper. New York: State University of New York Press, 1992. d

Sears, J. "Alston and Everetta: Too Risky for School?" In *At-Risk Students*, edited by R. Donmoyer and R. Kos. New York: State University of New York Press, 1993.

Shernoff, M. "Family Therapy for Lesbian and Gay Clients." *Social Work* 29, no. 4 (1984): 393-96.

Slater, B . "Essential Issues in Working with Lesbian and Gay Male Youths." *Professional Psychology: Research and Practice* 19, no. 2 (1988): 226-35.

Smith, B., ed. *Some Girls: A Black Feminist Anthology*. New York: Kitchen Table, Women of Color Press, 1983.

Stewart, J. "What Non-Gay Therapists Need to Know to Work with Gay and Lesbian Clients." *Practice Digest* 7, no. 1 (1984): 28-32.

Stover, D. "The At-Risk Kids Schools Ignore." *Executive Educator* 14, no. 3 (1992): 28-31.

Summerford, S. "The Public Library: Offensive by Design." *Public Libraries* 26, no. 2 (1987): 60-62.

Tabbert, B. "Battling Over Books: Freedom and Responsibility Are Tested." *Emergency Librarian* 16, no. 1 (1988): 9-13.

Teague, J. "Issues Relating to the Treatment of Adolescent Lesbians and Homosexuals." *Journal of Mental Health Counseling* 14, no. 4 (1992): 422-39.

Turner, P.; Scadden, L.; and Harris, M. "Parenting in Gay and Lesbian Families." Paper presented at the First Annual Future of Parenting Symposium, Chicago, March 1985.

Vazquez, R. "(No Longer) Sleeping with the Enemy." *Empathy* 3, no. 1 (1992): 90-91.

Weeks, R.; Derdeyn, A.; and Langman, M. "Two Cases of Children of Homosexuals." *Child Psychiatry and Human Development* 6, no. 1 (1975): 26-32.

Weinberg, G. *Society and the Healthy Homosexual*. New York: St. Martin's Press, 1972.

Wilhoite, M. *Daddy's Roommate*. Boston: Alyson, 1990.

Wilson, D. "The Open Library." *English Journal* 43, no. 7 (1984): 60-63.

Wolf, T. "Marriages of Bisexual Men." *Journal of Homosexuality* 4 (1985): 135-48.

Wyers, N. *Lesbian and Gay Spouses and Parents: Homosexuality in the Family*. Portland, Ore.: Portland State University School of Social Work, 1984.

Wyers, N. "Homosexuality in the Family: Lesbian and Gay Spouses." *Social Work* 32, no. 2 (1987): 143-48.

Zera, D. "Coming of Age in a Heterosexist World: The Development of Gay and Lesbian Adolescents." *Adolescence* 27, no. 108 (1992): 849-54.

Part Four
Responses

Teaching Under Siege: Lesbian and Gay Educators in Colorado and Oregon

by Rita M. Kissen

In 1992 Colorado voters approved a ballot referendum preventing homosexuals from pursuing legal protection against discrimination. That year, a similar referendum was rejected in Oregon. Two years later, the Oregon referendum was resurrected and again defeated, although this time by a narrower margin. At the same time, Idaho voters barely rejected an anti-gay initiative, while attempts to limit the rights of lesbians and gays in other states failed only because their promoters did not secure the required number of petition signatures. In every case, these attempts to deny the legal rights of lesbians and gay men have singled out gay teachers.

Why teachers? For one thing, targeting teachers allows the proponents of anti-gay legislation to manipulate parents' legitimate concerns for the safety of their children by evoking long-standing myths about pedophilia. For another, the identification of lesbians and gay men with sexuality — as if that were the only aspect of their identity — plays into the public debate over sex education, a debate that, in turn, touches on Americans' deepest anxieties and repressions. Accordingly, lesbian and gay teachers have become the primary target of the Radical Right's newest weapon, the ballot initiative. And "weapon" is the operant term; if there is one thing that advocates of lesbian and gay equality and their enemies agree on, it is that there is a war under way, and America's schools are the battleground.

In 1994 and 1995 I traveled to Colorado and Oregon to meet with lesbian, gay, and bisexual teachers and activists who had lived through Amendment 2, Ballot Measure 9, and Ballot Measure 13. As a teacher educator, I wanted to understand what happens when teachers become the focus of concerted political efforts to vilify them. As a veteran of a successful 1992 campaign to uphold a gay rights ordinance in Portland, Maine, I was familiar with debates within the gay community over image and disclosure and was eager to see how these issues played out when the stakes were highest. And, as the parent of a lesbian teacher, I felt a personal relationship to educators who had been living and working under siege for at least half a dozen years.

> *. . . rumors began to fly about the opposition's secret tactics against teachers.*

The Colorado Experience

The story of Colorado's Amendment 2 begins in 1990, the year the Colorado Springs Human Relations Council began reworking its charter. John Miller*, a faculty member at the University of Colorado in Colorado Springs, "somewhat optimistically" organized a small group of gay men and lesbians who presented a recommendation to the Human Relations Council that sexual orientation be included in human rights protections for the citizens of Colorado Springs. The Human Relations Council approved the recommendation and brought it to the full City Council, which held public hearings where, in John's words, "there were hundreds of basically fundamentalist Christians who were called out by their pastors to do witness. And that was the beginning of the Amendment 2 controversy."

Eventually, the anti-gay leadership joined forces as the Coalition for Family Values, led by a Colorado Springs car salesman named Will Perkins.

---

*I have tried to honor both the need for safety and the desire for authenticity by adhering as closely as possible to the wishes of the teachers themselves in matters of identification. Teachers who chose to use a pseudonym are referred to with quotation marks the first time they are mentioned; those who chose to use their own names are referred to without quotation marks. In a few cases, when I have quoted community leaders or others with relatively public identities, I have used first and last names at their request.

Political and financial inspiration came from Focus on the Family, a conservative religious foundation housed in a fortress-like complex north of Colorado Springs.

By 1992, proponents had gathered enough signatures to place their initiative on the ballot. Amendment 2 barred state agencies from enforcing any provisions protecting lesbians and gay men from discrimination, thereby nullifying civil rights ordinances already in effect in Denver, Boulder, and Aspen and precluding the passage of anti-discrimination legislation in the rest of the state.

Like others in the gay community, lesbian and gay teachers were involved in the struggle against Amendment 2 from the beginning. Those who felt the need to hide their sexual orientation at school found the challenge especially difficult. Like "Bill," an elementary school principal in Colorado Springs, they wondered, "How am I going to take some position on this without also trying to. . . be an activist and be up on stage?"

Others who were more visible began organizing among their colleagues as well as in the gay community at large. In Colorado Springs, teacher advocacy centered on a support group for gay and lesbian educators that had begun in 1990. In Denver, the Teachers Group had been meeting for more than 15 years, first as a social organization for gay men and later as a lesbian and gay advocacy group. Within both groups, teachers disagreed on how open their activity ought to be. Denver middle school teacher Tracy Phariss, one of the most public figures in the community of gay and lesbian educators, was impatient with those who wanted to maintain a low profile:

> A lot of teachers said, "Well, we shouldn't be getting involved in this because this is a political activity." . . . They would still volunteer their time but it would be . . . not as a teacher, just as a gay man. They have difficulty in correlating the two. You can't just be a teacher. You have to be a teacher and a gay man. You can't just be a gay man. You're also a teacher by heart.

As the campaign heated up, schools and classrooms reflected the charged atmosphere of the world outside. Barbara, a teacher in Colorado Springs, recalled:

It's very hard when you have students that you like and that you're trying to, you know, mold and direct toward a good life and so forth. They said things that were so horrid. . . . I had. . . one kid say, "Well, faggots should all be hanged." . . . Most of them said that they did not know anyone who was a gay person.

It was even harder to hear the anti-gay rhetoric of colleagues and administrators. Michelle, a Denver middle school teacher, remembered:

walking into the teachers' lounge and two of the men were discussing Amendment 2 and one guy was saying, "Oh, I think it's right. I think these people should be taken out and shot, and blah, blah, blah," and I turned around and I said, "You know, you work with one. You want to take me out and shoot me?" and they got real quiet. I said, "Thank you very much," and walked out.

For Lyn Boudreau, an elementary school teacher in Colorado Springs, coming out to colleagues was a happier experience:

I found myself being more and more open about talking about the issue. . . . Sometimes you get this look from other teachers. . . . Most of all, though, I would say the reaction was positive.

Some teachers, like Tracy Phariss, were able to disclose their identity to students and found that students who knew their teacher was gay were more likely to support the defeat of Amendment 2. "They didn't understand that [it] would have cost me my job," he explained. "But when I was telling the kids that, that really made a difference because they did care for me."

In addition to conflicts over visibility, teachers' struggles to defeat Amendment 2 reflected divisions in the gay community as a whole. There were regional tensions between urban Denver and conservative Colorado Springs and mistrust between gay men and lesbians. Teachers of color struggled to build coalitions with the mainly white leadership of EPOC (Equal Protection/Colorado) and the teachers groups within it. Like Dan, a Hispanic Denver middle school teacher, they sometimes resented being treated as "a token." Yet throughout the campaign, many lesbian and gay teachers worked hard to overcome these divisions.

One of their most important strategies was to involve the Colorado Education Association in the campaign and the court challenge that followed. As a branch of the National Education Association, one of the nation's two largest teacher unions, the CEA had both a local and a national perspective, as well as a commitment to equity reflected in the NEA's stands on a variety of civil rights issues. Traci Collins, a lesbian faculty member at Colorado Mountain College, was elected to the CEA board of directors in April 1992. She spent the spring and summer of 1992 making sure that literature went out to the CEA locals, knocking on doors, and generally making the implications of Amendment 2 clear to the teacher community at large. At the 1992 state convention, she lobbied for a resolution putting CEA on record against Amendment 2, a proposal that provoked a noisy and emotional debate as teachers affiliated with the Christian Right (many of them from Colorado Springs) raised the familiar specters of "special rights" and pedophilia. In the end, the resolution passed by an overwhelming margin (more than 95%, according to Collins' estimate).

Before long, rumors began to fly about the opposition's secret tactics against teachers. Virtually everyone I met was convinced that Focus on the Family had collected lists of lesbian and gay educators. Bill was in a good position to assess the reliability of the rumor because of his role as a school administrator. "I called some friends in the administration to say, 'Have you heard this rumor, and is it true?' and the denial of it was so blatant that it almost felt like, yeah, there was some truth to what was going on," he said.

Curt, a high school teacher, heard about the witch hunts at a meeting in Colorado Springs. "The rumor was that. . . they were going out of their way to find out who the unmarried teachers over thirty were, both male and female, and they were going to target them," recalled Curt. Back in more liberal Denver, a high school teacher named Tim recalled that representatives of Coloradans for Family Values "were calling school buildings and asking secretaries for the names and addresses of all single teachers."

Whatever the extent of the witch hunt, it appears to have backfired. Frank, a Colorado Springs teacher who worked with a group called Citizen's Project, reported that when his organization confronted Focus on the Family with allegations that they had been collecting names of gay teachers, "they denied it, and there was never any proof that they'd done it. . . . When it was reported, there was a such a negative reaction that I think . . . whoever it was stopped."

Election Day 1992 was a traumatic moment for Colorado's lesbian and gay educators. In Denver, "Leslie" joined about 4,000 others at the Event Center to watch the returns. Early figures from Denver and Boulder made it seem that Amendment 2 was going down to defeat. Leslie recounted the changing emotions:

> Twenty minutes later or so. . . as more precincts were counted, now it's even. . . . And then as the night wears on, it becomes real clear that it's going to pass; and at that point it got kind of scary. People were either incredibly angry or like somebody had died — in total grief.

Following the news, a spontaneous march took place at the Capitol. Michelle recalled:

> I was at the big rally. . . . Maybe 150 or 200 people gathered and marched. . . . It was frightening. You could feel the fear and, yes, right after the election there were people being attacked. . . . It happened . . . even in Denver.

In Colorado Springs, the gay response was more muted but no less intense. Many gathered in the park for a candlelight vigil where, as "Rodney" recalled, "It was very emotional. . . . I wasn't angry, I was just depressed, and just very, very sad."

Wednesday, 4 November 1992, was a regular school day for lesbian and gay educators in Colorado, as it was for everyone else in the nation. In Denver, Tracy Phariss wore a pink and black triangle to school. Across town, in her junior high school classroom, Leslie felt "totally numb . . . just [going] through the motions of the day and trying not to talk about it to anybody," until a student teacher came into her room during a break. Leslie recalled:

> I'm putting things [away] and then he walks up to me and he turns around and he says, "I'm so sorry." And I just lost it. . . . He put his arms around me, you know, and he just hugged me for a long time and I just cried.

In Colorado Springs, Rick's straight colleagues "came up to me and put their arm around me or put their arm on my shoulder or something and said, 'We know it's tough, but we're here for you'." Lyn Boudreau's principal gave her "a big shake of the hand, and her eyes filled with tears. She said, 'Thank you for what you did'."

Looking back from a vantage point of two years, lesbian and gay teachers agreed that Amendment 2 changed their lives forever. Tracy Phariss believes it "devastated our community. Teachers went further into the closet than I've ever seen. I've seen teachers who [were] just coming out slam the door and go the other way." Yet when I asked him about the net effect of the campaign on gay teachers, Phariss was sure that on balance Amendment 2 was a spur to greater visibility rather than less. "I would say personally around the state . . . that more teachers came out, but I would say that they're in the metropolitan areas. In the rural areas they went more in." He added that he personally knew three rural teachers who had been fired, with Amendment 2 given as the explicit reason:

[Colorado's] Amendment 2 was a spur to greater visibility rather than less.

> They were so scared because they still lived in the community, they weren't willing to do anything, press charges. . . . One of them even was a non-probationary teacher and they broke the contract when they fired him, but he wasn't willing to do anything.

Being fired was not always the reason why teachers hesitated to come out in Colorado. In Denver, where most teachers doubted that they would be fired for being gay, the issue was one of "credibility with kids," as Leslie put it. "I live in a homophobic society which creates impressions, and if those kids come in, those impressions that they have could cause us to lose them as an audience."

Yet most teachers in both Colorado Springs and Denver saw Amendment 2 as a wake-up call, rather than a reason to retreat into the closet. Gary, a Colorado Springs junior high school teacher, declared, "For me personally, it has made me almost more out than I was before, just because it's such a stupid thing, you know." Tim, who started a high school support group for gay youth in the midst of the campaign, agreed that Amendment 2 had made him "think more about other people and less about myself, and more about what I can do as an individual."

229

Traci Collins remains cautiously optimistic: "I was just amazed that we came as close as we did [53% to 47%]. . . . Anyone who follows state politics in Colorado, and particularly looks at the composition of the Colorado state legislature, knows what a politically conservative state this is."

The Oregon Experience

Portland, Oregon, like Denver, is a city with a reputation for tolerance. Teachers in the Portland area had been organizing even before Measure 9 found its way to the 1992 ballot, both in the Cascade Union of Educators, a social group that revolved around potlucks and get-togethers, and in the more politically oriented Educators for Equity, an organization founded in 1992.

The activists' first project was to get sexual orientation into the language of the Portland teachers' contract. For this they turned to the Oregon Education Association, the statewide affiliate of the NEA. Like its Colorado counterpart, the OEA allied itself with its lesbian and gay constituency. By the end of the 1992 bargaining period, sexual orientation protection had been written into Portland teachers' contracts, though efforts to include domestic partnership benefits had not yet succeeded.

Just as the OEA was achieving its first victories against discrimination based on sexual orientation, a coalition of right-wing religious and political groups, called the Oregon Citizen's Alliance, started collecting signatures to place a question on the 1992 ballot intended to deny civil rights protection to anyone known or perceived to be lesbian or gay. The Oregon initiative went further than Colorado's Amendment 2 by equating homosexuality with sadomasochism and pedophilia as "abnormal, wrong, unnatural and perverse" and barring the state from doing anything to "encourage" such behavior. Educators for Equity and the OEA shifted their energies to defeating Ballot Measure 9.

During the summer of 1992, Educators for Equity members worked with the OEA to arrange meetings with the directors of the statewide "No on Nine" campaign. "At that point it became survival oriented," recalled Barb, a founder of Educators for Equity. "The spring was exciting and affirming, and then it was into total survival."

Oregon teachers, like their colleagues in Colorado, found the challenge to put themselves on the line empowering at the same time that it was frightening. "When we started feeling backed up against the wall . . . it sort of just kind of all came together," explained Karen, a Portland elementary school teacher active in Educators for Equity. She continued:

> It's like I knew I was a lesbian before I was a teacher and I'd be one after I was a teacher. It was the thing that was with me really to stay, and I felt that I had to be true to that first. . . . I . . . actually called the Oregon Citizens Alliance to thank them for the courage that they had given me to come out at my school and to relatives.

As in Colorado, being "out" in school meant more than just stating one's sexual orientation. Ron, the co-founder of Educators for Equity, recalled:

> It was a very tense period. . . . They wanted to put us in the same classification as people who have sex with animals and . . . corpses. . . . [Measure 9] attacked me to the core in such a great way, I realized for the first time in my life that, yeah, there were some issues I'd be willing to die for.

As the campaign heated up, so did the atmosphere in schools and classrooms. "Annette," who has taught high school in Portland for 21 years, experienced both support and hostility from her colleagues. One evening, she attended a school board meeting where a vote was taken to oppose Measure 9. The next day, the principal told Annette that she had seen her on the news. Annette recalled:

> I said, "Yes, I was there at the school board meeting." She said, "Well, there's no room for hate at this school." . . . She was trying to make me feel safe and I really appreciated that. . . . On the other hand, I was in the Xerox room that day and . . . a secretary . . . came up to me and she said, "I saw you on the news last night. What were you doing there? Why would you be there? I couldn't understand why you would be there. You know, gay people? Homosexuals?" I said, "Well . . . I'm gay. I'm a lesbian." She said, "You are?" . . . And then she said, "I have a cousin that's

231

gay . . . and we still have her over." [I thought], "You still have her over, isn't that great."

Mike, a Portland elementary school teacher, found that wearing and carrying "No on Nine" pins "was kind of an opportunity to be out without having to say it, just to be myself, really." Ron admitted that he felt uneasy wearing a button to school for the first few weeks of the campaign; but as the election drew closer, "it was really important to do it."

"Will," a teacher at an inner-city Portland high school, found his students generally supportive,

> except for those born-again Christian kids. . . . They said, "Well you know, it's a sin against God and blah-blah-blah and we love the homosexuals but we hate homosexuality," and, you know, the stock line. They were eaten alive by the other students in the class.

. . . lesbian and gay teachers will not disappear.

Martha recalled a moment when a student in her room wearing a "Yes on Nine" button was challenged by another student, who said, "Why are you wearing that? . . . My aunt is a lesbian and she's just a person, and you shouldn't be wearing that."

Whatever their experiences, Oregon teachers, like those in Colorado, felt increasingly exposed during the campaign. Many chose to affirm their visibility. Barb brought her partner to the faculty Christmas party for the first time. "It was at our principal's house, so I felt very nervous about it, but I felt like I wanted to do that. . . . It was the year of everything revolved around people knowing I was gay."

And, like their Colorado counterparts, Oregon teachers were grateful for the support of allies who made their ordeal more bearable. Karen remembered a straight teacher who responded to students' homophobic remarks with a three-day unit on gay issues, complete with guest speakers. "Sue," a Portland middle school teacher, came out to the only teacher of color in her building after a racist comment appeared on the school's E-mail. The woman responded, "I'll tell you what. If you fight mine, I'll fight yours."

Speculation over the outcome of the referendum increased as the election approached. As in Colorado, polls predicted the referendum's defeat by a comfortable margin. Afterward, as Karen recounted, relief over the victory was tempered by anxiety.

> We were all really upset and scared about how close it was [56% to 44%]. You know, it's easy to live in the city [Portland] in Multnomah County where it was defeated . . . three to one or something, but to realize once you cross the city line . . .

Both Portland area gay teachers groups resolved to continue meeting after the election. Educators for Equity shifted their work to domestic partnership benefits for lesbian and gay teachers, and CUE returned to its original focus as a social group. But no one in the gay community had time to rest for long.

The Oregon Citizen's Alliance had learned from its initial defeat. By the time Measure 13 appeared on the 1994 ballot, it had been renamed the "Minority Status and Child Protection Act," and, as Ron put it,

> toned down a lot. . . . Just on the surface, you know, basically it was saying do you think that homosexuals as a minority group should have special rights? And the other thing was, is, do you think children need to be protected? . . . So it was brilliant, but it was deceptively brilliant.

Like his colleagues, Ron felt "exhausted" by this time:

> Along with everybody else that I knew of, [I] felt like I had been beaten with a two by four for the past two years and hardly had the energy to stand up and do anything in the face of it. But I did. I got active.

Like Ron, Mike was torn between his commitment to activism and his exhaustion after the Measure 9 campaign:

> Part of the time I was maybe in denial [thinking] that this is not going to make it on to the ballot. . . . Then the other side of me would come back: definitely you don't want it to pass because think of all the kids who would be seeing that this many people in the State of Oregon think [gay people] are abnormal, that they're not good human beings.

Martha, who remained active in CUE, admitted, "It felt different for me. I knew I couldn't engage emotionally in the same way." Karen summed up the dispirited mood:

> You know, we've been to this fund-raiser, we've been to this auction, we've seen these people, we've given our money, they've given their money, we've said these things, and we'll all be at that same auction again and we'll all be at the same house party, and we'll all be giving our same money — that gets old. To get what? To get not a whole lot. . . . Not even to win anything.

Still, many gay teachers found that they were able to come out more during the Measure 13 campaign than they had during Measure 9. Karen, for example, said she "talked about my involvement with the campaign more. . . . This time if people said, 'What are you doing this weekend?' I'd say, 'Well, I'm canvassing for No on Thirteen,' or 'I'm phone banking for No on Thirteen'."

Sue, who had been involved with both CUE and Educators for Equity before Measure 9, was part of a group that brought the NAMES Quilt to her school in February 1993. For Sue, the quilt had personal as well as political significance; her brother had died of AIDS exactly five years earlier.

As soon as word got out that the quilt was coming, a husband and wife team in her building, who had been active in the "Yes on Nine" campaign (Sue calls them "Mr. and Mrs. OCA"), began agitating in the community. Sue recalled:

> We had parents coming in and the principal was in after school because they were so upset about the quilt being here. And the. . . husband . . . was taking pictures of the quilt and sending it to OCA headquarters, saying, "This is the homosexual agenda in our building, it's happening here."

At the unfolding ceremony, Sue gave a brief talk to the assembled students, parents, teachers, and community members. "It was wonderful," Sue recalled. "I mean, 500, 600 kids packed into that gym. And it was the quietest I've ever heard that many middle-schoolers. . . . It was really an incredible ceremony."

Some Oregon teachers reported that harassment against them increased during the second campaign. Like Annette, they felt Measure 13 gave people "a green light to . . . express their hatred for gay people." Teachers in rural areas felt particularly insecure during the 1994 campaign. Although most of the teachers I interviewed live in and around Portland, several had friends and colleagues outside the city and could speak about the climate in the rest of the state.

Yet even in Portland, where their contract language meant that most teachers had little fear of actually losing their jobs, many felt insecure. Will, whose students were supportive, admitted that this support did not make him feel more safe:

> I guess I would want to. . . teach in a place that was 100% supportive of me being gay. I don't want people who are just going to tolerate me being gay. . . . When I talk to kids now and I look in their eyes . . . there's a lot of joy and love, and that's really why I'm there. . . . If that were to change because of who I am, then I don't think I'd want to teach anymore.

Carolyn, another high school teacher, agreed: "What do you fear? I don't know what you fear. . . . I guess it would be . . . being accused or of being proven unprofessional."

When Measure 13 went down to defeat in November 1994, gay teachers were relieved; but they also were alarmed by the narrowness of their victory — only two percentage points. For Mike, the narrow margin was part of a bigger picture: "Around the country . . . more Republicans were winning, and this whole package was coming together. . . . When the numbers started coming in, it was kind of like reality hit."

Since the 1994 election, both CUE and Educators for Equity have lost some momentum. When I interviewed Ron in January 1995, a mailing had just gone out to the Educators for Equity membership proposing that the group disband. But Ron believes that the work will go on: "What I hope will happen next is that. . . there will be a gay and lesbian caucus that will form within the Oregon Education Association. . . . It's moving more to the mainstream, you know."

Unlike Educators for Equity, CUE still is meeting, though it has resumed its social character. Martha, who is no longer in a leadership role, feels that such meetings help to build alliances among people in different schools and different buildings, alliances that could be mobilized for grassroots organizing when the next political crisis erupts.

Despite their weariness, many gay teachers in Oregon find reasons for optimism. Like Barb, they take comfort from the fact that Measure 13 was, in fact, defeated. "When Thirteen went down, it didn't go down by a lot, but it went down again. In such a conservative national climate it still went down. And so I think that's encouraging."

As of this writing, anti-gay ballot initiatives are being formulated in states from Maine to Washington. At the same time, the U.S. Supreme Court has agreed to hear the Colorado case sometime in the fall of 1995. If the High Court declares Amendment 2 unconstitutional, as civil rights advocates hope, the position of lesbian and gay teachers in Oregon and Colorado, and everywhere else, will be strengthened immeasurably. But even if the Court upholds Amendment 2, fueling ballot campaigns in other states, lesbian and gay teachers will not disappear. Most of the gay teachers who survived the ballot campaigns in Colorado and Oregon are determined to stay in teaching. They have begun to connect with other lesbian and gay educators, not only in their home states but all over the country. Like Colorado's Traci Collins, they take the long view:

> I guess I'm optimistic. It may not sound that way, [but] I don't think you get rights without controversy and without struggle, and I think we're reaching that kind of momentum where . . . the consensus is that we shouldn't be discriminated against, and that is an exhilarating feeling.

Traci's words can serve as a hopeful comment on the Colorado and Oregon campaigns, as well as on the current struggles being waged by lesbian and gay teachers across the country. Near the end of our conversation, she reflected on the meaning of her work with the CEA during the Amendment 2 campaign. Her comment is a fitting summary:

> In many ways I think the radical right is doing us a favor by making the nation confront this issue, because I think that if the nation truly confronts this issue, we'll win and they'll lose. It won't happen instantly, but it is happening as time goes on. And that's what we're working for.

Project 10: A School-Based Outreach to Gay and Lesbian Youth*

by Virginia Uribe

This decade is emerging as the "gay nineties" because of the increased visibility of gay and lesbian issues in the media and in the public consciousness. As one of the major institutions in society, the education system is facing one of its most pressing challenges — the acknowledgment of gay and lesbian youth as a significant part of the total school population. Because their existence is less visible than other minorities, youthful homosexuals are often ignored. Crossing every boundary of race, religion and class, they have sat through years of public school education where their identities have been overlooked, denied, or abused. They have been quiet due to their own fear and sense of isolation, as well as the failure of their parents and of adult gay men and women to be their advocates. The result has been the creation of a group of youngsters within our schools who are at significantly high risk of dropping out of school.

In 1989 the United States Department of Health and Human Services issued a report on teen suicide that noted the startling fact that as many as 30% of all teenage suicides may be linked to conflict over homosexuality.[1] This

*This article first appeared in *The High School Journal* 77, nos. 1 and 2 (October-November 1993/December-January 1994): 108-12. Reprinted with permission of the author and the publisher.]

information alone should prompt educators to examine existing attitudes toward homosexuality, the effect of these attitudes on both the gay and non-gay population, and how such attitudes are contrary to the public school mission of teaching all children respect for individual diversity.

Negative biases have often been espoused by critical persons within the homosexual child's educational milieu, such as school principals, teachers, coaches, counselors and peers.[2] To a varying degree, these prevalent negative attitudes are byproducts of the conscious and unconscious fears and reactions that have come to be known as homophobia, the irrational fear of homosexuals or of the subject of homosexuality.

Project 10 — A Model School Program

Project 10 began in 1984 as a way of addressing the underserved needs of gay and lesbian students in the Los Angeles Unified School District. A model program was developed by Dr. Virginia Uribe, a counselor at Fairfax High School, one of the 52 senior high schools in the LAUSD. The focus of the model is education, reduction of verbal and physical abuse, suicide prevention, and dissemination of accurate AIDS information. The method by which this is carried out is through workshops for teachers, counselors, and other support personnel and through support groups set up on each senior high school campus for students dealing with sexual orientation issues. The goal of the support groups is to improve self-esteem and to provide affirmation for students suffering the effects of stigmatization and discrimination based on sexual orientation.

Project 10 groups average 10-12 students at a given time. All races and family backgrounds are represented. About 65% of the students are males. Students are informed of the existence of Project 10 groups through signs in the counselor's office, word of mouth, and referrals by counselors or teachers. Participation is completely voluntary. Absolute confidentiality of groups is maintained, and no one is permitted in the group except the participants and the facilitators. Usually there is one male and one female who serve as co-facilitators. Some of the facilitators are gay or lesbian; most are not. All the facilitators operate on a volunteer basis.

The labels *gay* and *lesbian* are generic. Actually, the groups have many students who identify as bisexual, transgender, or unsure. It is not the phi-

It is not the philosophy of the program to impose labels, but rather to provide a "safe space" for these young people to talk freely.

losophy of the program to impose labels, but rather to provide a "safe space" for these young people to talk freely. We ask that all adults be trained through workshops before they agree to be facilitators, and they must be nonjudgmental with regard to sexual orientation.

The support groups make up the heart of the Project program. Most students in these groups have social, family, or personal problems that affect their academic work. In addition to dealing with issues of sexual orientation, the counselors/facilitators provide counseling with issues such as staying off drugs and alcohol, avoiding high-risk sexual behavior, getting jobs, staying in school, and going to college. When appropriate, facilitators suggest outside agencies that may be able to provide additional services. Most of the support groups meet once a week, sometimes after school, sometimes during the lunch hour, and sometimes during the school day.

Without question, the disclosure of homosexuality by a gay or lesbian child is a traumatic event.

Testimonials from the students themselves indicate that the support groups are valuable and empowering for them. Success also is measured in terms of improved attendance and academic performance, improved relationships with primary family members, and by the number of males who agree to attend AIDS education programs sponsored by local human service organizations.

A small number of people, mostly from organized groups, have criticized the Project 10 program. They characterize it as a recruitment program, that it promotes homosexuality, and that homosexuality is a subject that should not be dealt with in school. Opponents stage periodic demonstrations at the Los Angeles Board of Education.

The Project 10 model of education and schoolsite support groups has been sought out by educators throughout the United States and Canada. As can be seen, it is a fluid model, adaptable to individual school and district needs. In its most ideal form, the Project 10 model consists of 1) a district resource center; 2) a paid coordinator for the program; 3) ongoing workshops to train counselors, teachers, and other staff members on issues of institutional homophobia and the special needs of gay and lesbian youth; 4) development of trained on-site school teams to whom students can go for information and support; 5) assistance to librarians in developing fiction and nonfiction on gay/lesbian subjects; 6) enforcement of nondiscrimination clauses, antislur resolutions, and codes of behavior with regard to name-calling; 7) advocacy for lesbian and gay student rights through commissions, task forces, PTAs and community outreach programs; and 8) networking with community agencies, parents, education organizations, and teachers unions.

What About Parents?

Discrimination on the basis of sexual orientation often is compounded by economic disadvantage.

Without question, the disclosure of homosexuality by a gay or lesbian child is a traumatic event. Family relationships are a major concern for the adolescent, and a great deal of anxiety often is associated with whether or not to "come out" to parents and, if so, how it should be done. There is no formula for this process, and the ways in which children disclose are as varied as the individuals themselves.

The fear of rejection or disapproval is ever present. For some young people the threat of expulsion from the home is very real. In many instances, exposure is forced; parents discover their child's homosexuality by accident, and the young person is pressed into revealing the fact prior to adequate preparation.

The strategy of deception that characterizes the development of lesbian and gay socialization distorts almost all relationships, including family relationships. The adolescent may attempt to develop or maintain and create an increasing sense of isolation. The adolescent realizes that his or her membership in the family is based on a lie. Even in their homes, the youngsters are forced to act a role. Distancing becomes a mechanism of survival for lesbian and gay adolescents with the fear that their parents will discover their secret.

Ineffective communication, poor self-esteem, and unresolved grief and anger often complicate "coming out." Frequently, misinformation about homosexuality, religious beliefs, and homophobia can have a negative influence in the disclosure process.

Educators should understand that when a child "comes out," the parent must also "come out" and yield all their heterosexual expectations for that child. This process can be very difficult and can take months or years. Parents typically pass through stages of denial and anger. Some reach a grudging acceptance of things they cannot change. Others educate themselves and begin to accept their children with the unconditional love that is so desperately needed. One group that is extremely helpful for parents going through this process is an organization called Parents and Friends of Lesbians and Gays (PFLAG), which has more than 200 chapters in the United States and Canada.[3] Educators should familiarize themselves with their local chapters and make use of their services.

Gay and Lesbian Teens of Color

The various cultures and races reflected in the United States also are reflected in the lesbian and gay population. Such adolescents face the prospect of living their lives within three rigidly defined and strongly independent communities: the lesbian and gay community, their ethnic or racial community, and the society at large. Each community fulfills basic needs that often are imperiled if such communities were to be visibly integrated. A common result is the constant effort to maintain a manner of living that keeps the three communities separate, a process that leads to increased isolation, depression, and anger centered on the fear of being separated from all support systems, including the family.

Discrimination on the basis of sexual orientation often is compounded by economic disadvantage. A person of color, or a woman of any color, is more easily subjected to discrimination policies. Further, unemployment rates are higher among some minority groups, adding the burden of poverty, drug abuse, and alcohol to the quality of interaction among lesbian and gay persons of color.

The upholding of negative stereotyping and the practice of discrimination against lesbians and gays places the ethnic gay man and lesbian as the least desirable combination for acceptance and assimilation. A hierarchy — suggesting preferences for whites over Latins, over blacks, over Asians, over American Indians or any combination of these except for whites — defines and complicates the level and intensity of discrimination. This endless downward spiral continues when one introduces other variables, such as gender, sex role behavior, physical disabilities, shades of skin color, age, religious affiliation, and other variables.

As with parent issues, school personnel need to recognize the special issues that exist among minority lesbians and gays and should familiarize themselves with any community resources that may exist.

Students on the verge of adulthood have a right to seek information about current social issues and to develop critical skills based on scientific evidence and social justice, rather than on myth and ignorance.

241

Setting Up a Gay Friendly Curriculum

Gay and lesbian students are perhaps the most underserved students in the entire education system.

When we talk about a "gay friendly" curriculum, it is important to define what we mean. A special course in gay and lesbian studies probably won't happen in the near future in a high school setting. What we can try to do, however, is to encourage teachers to include gay and lesbian topics in their individual classes whenever it is relevant and appropriate. For example, there are many occasions in a health education class when the subject of homosexuality will arise; the same is true in history, psychology, political science, and art classes. In almost any class where there is a lot of interaction, gay and lesbian topics will come up if the students feel that it is safe to discuss them. In this connection, there are two problems. First, many teachers feel awkward or ill-prepared to discuss homosexuality; but it should be kept in mind that a lot of clinical knowledge isn't necessary — most if the issues are with attitude. Second, some people feel that if they discuss homosexuality in anything but negative terms, they will be accused of "condoning" or "promoting" it. This assertion should be placed in the irrational category to which it belongs. Gay and lesbian topics are in the newspapers, magazines, on radio, TV dramas, talk shows, and news programs. In short, they are everywhere. Students on the verge of adulthood have a right to seek information about current social issues and to develop critical skills based on scientific evidence and social justice, rather than on myth and ignorance.

Related to curriculum is the question of setting up a gay-oriented club on a high school campus. This is different from a support group, though both could exist on a campus. We had some experience in doing this at Fairfax High School, where a group of gay and non-gay students chartered a club called the Harvey Milk Club. The purpose of the club was educational. The club had a constitution that followed the format of all other school clubs, and it was open to anyone. The setting was not confidential, and the issues discussed were societal rather than personal. Films were shown, and various speakers addressed the group. The club was involved in such school activities as the Club Fair, and they did fundraisers from time to time. The administration was somewhat skittish about the club, and they sought advice from the district lawyers, who could find no reason for the Harvey Milk Club not to exist. It was not entirely a rosy picture. Many students didn't want to

242

come near a club that was identified as gay or lesbian even if it was open to everyone. When the main organizers graduated, the club stopped functioning. More recently, a coalition of private schools on the east coast has formed a Gay/ Straight Alliance, which exists successfully in several schools.[4]

Tips for School Administrators

In the current climate, administrators will at some time probably have to face a variety of gay- and lesbian-related situations. Examples include: teachers and students coming out of the closet; discussions of gay and lesbian issues in classrooms; teachers or students wanting to put up a display or a poster around gay and lesbian issues; counselors/teachers putting up hotline numbers, including those of gay and lesbian community centers; requests for speakers representing the gay and lesbian community; protests against ROTC programs or military recruiters on campus; instances of harassment against gay/lesbian teachers; same-sex couples wanting to go to the prom; and lesbian or gay parents.

The following suggestions have been drawn from real-life scenarios and may be helpful. Administrators should have a firm policy of nondiscrimination at their school site. Harassment against gay/lesbian teachers or students should not be tolerated, whether it be between students, students and teachers, or among teachers themselves. Disclosing one's sexual orientation is an option that teachers and students have if they choose to exercise it. Administrators should respect this option and protect both staff and students from a hostile environment to the extent that they can. Court cases have generally upheld the right of same-sex couples to attend school dances as long as their behavior is not disruptive. The conventional wisdom is "don't make a big issue out of it." Discussing gay and lesbian issues in a classroom is not the same as having a lesson on sex or reproduction. Teachers should be careful that the classroom discussion does not lapse into sexually explicit conversation. Finally, if a parent complaint should arise, ask them to put the complaint in writing, specifically stating their objections and the reasons for them. The administrator can then, calmly but firmly, review the complaint in light of the suggestions mentioned above.

Conclusion

Gay and lesbian students are perhaps the most underserved students in the entire education system. Prejudice and discrimination often interfere with their personal and academic development. Suicide rates are alarmingly high in this group, and this alone should prompt educators to examine existing attitudes toward homosexuality and the destructive effects that being stigmatized has on gay and lesbian youth. Supportive resources are meager, and therefore it is very important that faculty and staff workshops be instituted so that accurate information can begin to replace the myth and ignorance that surround the subject of homosexuality. The Project 10 model, developed in the Los Angeles Unified School District, is presented in this article as a model that can be replicated by any school or school district. Parent issues also must be examined, as well as making the school curriculum inclusive of gay and lesbian topics. Administrators must develop strategies for gay and lesbian situations that arise at their schools.

Above all, educators must commit themselves to the idea that the mission of public education is to serve all children, and that some children *are* gay and lesbian. To exclude these children, either by indifference or discrimination, is to perpetuate a system that is scientifically unsound and morally unjust.

Footnotes

1. P. Gibson, "Gay Male and Lesbian Youth Suicide," in *Report of the Secretary's Task Force on Youth Suicide*, edited by M. Feinleib (Washington, D.C.: U.S. Department of Health and Human Services, 1989).
2. R. Bidwell, "The Gay and Lesbian Teen: A Case of Denied Adolescence," *Journal of Pediatric Health Care* 2, no. 1 (1988): 3-8. J.P. DeCecco, *Bashers, Baiters, and Bigots: Homophobia in American Society* (New York: Harrington Park Press, 1984).
3. For materials and information about the nearest chapter, contact: Parents, Families, and Friends of Lesbians and Gays (PFLAG), P.O. Box 27605, Washington, DC 20038.
4. *You Are Not Alone: National Lesbian, Gay, and Bisexual Youth Organization Directory, Spring 1993.* Hetrick-Martin Institute, 2 Astor Place, New York, NY 10003.

How the IYG Helps
Gay Teens At Risk*

by Donovan R. Walling
and Christopher T. Gonzalez

"Hello, this is the IYG Youth Hotline."

"Uh, hi. Is this the hotline where people can . . . uh . . . call and talk to people?"

"Yes. My name is David. How are you tonight?"

"Well, I guess I'm not doing too good. You see, some kids beat me up today at school . . . and I'm real afraid to tell my parents why I got beat up. If they knew I was gay, they would kick me out."

Forty-five percent of gay males and 20% of lesbian females experience a verbal or physical assault in high school. Many are assaulted repeatedly. Twenty-eight percent drop out of school because of harassment over their sexual orientation (Remafedi 1987). Unable to openly express their feelings to peers or teachers and fearful of their parents' reaction to the disclosure of their sexual orientation, many homosexual adolescents desperately need a source of positive emotional support.

---

*This essay, written in 1993 and updated for this book, incorporates information graciously provided by the current IYG Executive Director, Jeffrey N. Werner. Christopher T. Gonzalez, the founding executive director of IYG, died on 5 May 1994.

The IYG Youth Hotline is the only nationwide, toll-free hotline specifically for gay teens. This peer-facilitated hotline offers an initial point of contact with a community support organization designed to help gay, lesbian, and bisexual teenagers combat alienation and isolation. The IYG (formerly Indianapolis Youth Group, prior to expanding to nine additional chapter sites across Indiana) offers gay, lesbian, and bisexual youth under age 21 social support and education designed to keep them from becoming at-risk statistics.

The organization has three formal goals: 1) to provide a safe, comfortable place for gay, lesbian, and bisexual youth to socialize and meet other gay, lesbian, and bisexual youth; 2) to provide a support system for these youth; and 3) to educate gay, lesbian, and bisexual youth in high-risk behavior reduction, including behaviors associated with HIV/AIDS infection and risks associated with substance abuse.

Being "Sexually Different"

In the words of researcher James T. Sears of the South Carolina Educational Policy Center, "[B]eing sexually different in a society of sexual sameness exacts a heavy psychological toll" (1991). That toll can lead "sexually different" teens to engage in behaviors that place them at risk not merely of academic failure but of social-emotional dysfunction, disease, and death.

According to some experts, between 5% and 15% of teens are gay or lesbian. Many gay teens "pass" — that is, act heterosexual — and parents, teachers, and peers never know that they are homosexual. More effeminate gay males or masculine-acting females are likely to be teased or harassed. The "closeted" nature of homosexuality offers few opportunities for positive expression, and thus homosexual and bisexual teens seldom are able to find positive role models, either adult or adolescent, to affirm their sexual orientation. As one researcher put it, "Growing up gay or lesbian is living daily with a terrible secret that no one must ever know" (Bidwell 1988).

Absent an affirming socialization process, many gay teens become disaffected. They exhibit low self-esteem, describe feelings of alienation, and reject (sometimes with hostility) the norms and expectations of school, home, and society. For example, many of the normal sexual rites of passage, such as dating activities, are denied to homosexual youngsters. Thus, without a

. . . many of the normal sexual rites of passage, such as dating activities, are denied to homosexual youngsters.

246

healthy pathway toward initial sexual exploration, gay teens sometimes resort to what Bidwell (1988) terms "the baths, bars, or bushes."

Anonymous sexual encounters in this era of the AIDS pandemic are extraordinarily risky. The highest number of new AIDS cases, according to the Centers for Disease Control and Prevention, is now among men and women between the ages of 20 and 29. Although the proportion of AIDS cases is rising among heterosexuals, about half of all AIDS cases are still the result of homosexual and bisexual contact. Because the dormancy period of the human immunodeficiency virus (HIV) can be up to 10 years, it takes little computation to conclude that homosexual and bisexual teenagers are significantly at risk of contracting this deadly disease. Indeed, many of those individuals in their 20s who are living with AIDS contracted HIV during adolescence.

For most teenagers, family support plays a crucial role in the development of a healthy self-image; but for homosexual adolescents, family support may be lacking. About half of gay and lesbian youth report being rejected by their parents because of their sexual orientation. One study found that 26% of gay youth are forced to leave home because of family conflicts over their sexual orientation (Remafedi 1987). The stories of homosexual and bisexual teens are often stories of runaways, throwaways, and suicides or attempted suicides.

A 1989 study by the U.S. Department of Health and Human Services found that gay and lesbian teens were far more likely than heterosexual teens to attempt suicide — up to eight times more likely for males. Gay and lesbian teens, that study found, accounted for 30% of all teen suicides. More recently, researchers from the Universities of Washington and Minnesota found that 41 of 137 gay or bisexual men interviewed said they had attempted suicide. About half of the respondents reported multiple attempts (Remafedi et al. 1991).

. . . when a teenager calls [the IYG hotline], he or she talks directly to another teen who has undergone a comprehensive 50-hour peer counselor/ educator training program.

Building a Support Organization

In 1987, two members of the Indianapolis Gay Switchboard, Christopher Gonzalez and Pat Jordan, were addressing a local university gay student group when they were asked about resources available to gay teens in the metropolitan area. The answer, they realized, was "none." That realization prompted a handful of gay and lesbian adults and adolescents to begin building a support organization — the IYG — that has become one of the nation's largest gay, lesbian, and bisexual youth projects.

Using a grant of $12,450 from the Indiana State Board of Health, the IYG was launched in 1988. By 1990, the group was setting up chapters across the state, making Indiana the only state with a network of community support for homosexual and bisexual youth. In July 1990, the IYG was recognized at the National Lesbian and Gay Health Conference in Washington, D.C., as a model program.

In March 1991, funded by a grant from the U.S. Conference of Mayors, the IYG developed the nation's first (and to date, only) toll-free peer counseling youth hotline. That means that when a teenager calls, he or she talks directly to another teen who has undergone a comprehensive 50-hour peer counselor/educator training program. The hotline, which also is accessible to the deaf and hearing impaired, offers peer counseling and information for youth under 21 with the goal of reducing feelings of isolation and rejection and increasing self-esteem.

A year later, in March 1992, the IYG received a grant of $50,000 from the Health Foundation of Greater Indianapolis to purchase an IYG Youth Center, which was occupied in August that year. The building is one of only three facilities in the United States dedicated solely to serving the needs of gay, lesbian, and bisexual young people.

Since that time, the IYG has grown steadily:

- The organization opened its first house for independent living, called the IYG Living Program, in November 1993. This resource provides transitional housing for 18- to 20-year-olds.
- A Street Outreach Counselor was added to the staff in December 1993, and a Street Outreach Team now works with street youth defined as "high-risk," providing information, education, and support.
- A Case Manager joined the staff in January 1994 to assist youth with individual needs in the areas of education, employment, and housing.
- In January 1995 a nurse practitioner was hired to provide health screenings, sexually transmitted disease testing, and holistic health education and counseling.

Today, more than 200 adult volunteers help implement IYG programs in 10 Indiana chapters.

A teenager's contact with IYG usually begins with a call to the Gay/Lesbian/Bisexual Youth Hotline: 1-800-347-TEEN (1-800-347-8336). For some teens, the hotline contact fulfills their need for information or simply to reach out to an understanding listener. For other youth, the IYG offers "face-to-face" services. Self-identified gay, lesbian, and bisexual adolescents can attend bi-weekly educational meetings, for example. The IYG also provides "toxic family" support groups to help youth deal with mental and physical abuse from family and peers, retreats to develop self-esteem and leadership skills, and peer-counseling training so that teens can be part of the support system for other adolescents.

The IYG offers a "safe haven" of social events, such as dances and roller-skating parties, which give gay, lesbian, and bisexual teens a safe place to socialize with one another. A drop-in center is open seven nights a week. Combating the isolation of being sexually different from the heterosexual majority, the IYG also coordinates a penpal network that matches youth under 21 with compatible penpals from across the United States. More than 350 youth nationwide are members of this network.

The IYG Ambassadors are teens who present workshops and panel discussions as an outreach information service to youth-serving agencies and community adolescents. Similarly, the IYG Interactive Theater presents skits to educate teens and adults about the needs of gay, lesbian, and bisexual youth — and to educate their peers about AIDS.

Since its inception in 1987, more than 5,000 Indiana youth have participated in "face-to-face" IYG programs. Tens of thousands from across the nation have called the Youth Hotline. Today, more than 200 adult volunteers help implement IYG programs in 10 Indiana chapters. Financial support is provided by individual contributions, the Centers for Disease Control and Prevention, the Indiana State Department of Health, and grants from other organizations and foundations.

The IYG success story has been featured in *Time* magazine, the *Advocate,* on "NBC News," Black Entertainment Television, and ABC's "20/20" news magazine. And the IYG model has been implemented and adapted in other communities.

Individuals interested in more information may contact IYG, P.O. Box 20716, Indianapolis, IN 46220, or call (317) 541-8726.

References

Bidwell, R.J. "The Gay and Lesbian Teen: A Case of Denied Adolescence." *Journal of Pediatric Health Care* 2 (1988).

Remafedi, G.J. "Homosexual Youth: A Challenge to Contemporary Society." *Journal of the American Medical Association* 258 (1987): 222-25.

Remafedi, G.J., et al. "Risk Factors for Attempted Suicide in Gay and Bisexual Youth." *Pediatrics* 87 (1991): 869

Sears, J.T. "Helping Students Understand and Accept Sexual Diversity." *Educational Leadership* (September 1991): 54-56.

"Together, for a Change": Lessons from Organizing the Gay, Lesbian, and Straight Teachers Network (GLSTN)

by Kevin Jennings

People sometimes ask me how the Gay, Lesbian, and Straight Teachers Network got started. The quick answer is, "I was lonely." That answer requires some explanation.

In 1985 I graduated from college and entered my first year of teaching at a private school in Providence, Rhode Island. The change of scenery was dramatic. I went from being an aggressively out undergraduate activist to being a closeted, traumatized young teacher who lived in dread of being fired by the openly homophobic administration of his school. I knew no other gay teachers, and this started me on a journey to find some kind of community. After two years I decided I had to get out, and I got a job teaching at Concord Academy, a private school located in suburban Boston. This time I knew that I had to be out to survive; the daily diminution of my self-esteem, the million white lies I had to tell to cover my tracks, the innumerable bitings-of-the-tongue that being closeted required, were simply out of the question for me. I was going to be truthful even if it cost me my job.

It didn't.

In the fall of 1988 I gave a chapel talk to the school — with all faculty and students present — in which I discussed being gay and what it had meant for my life. The response was electric, with students and colleagues hugging and embracing me all day long as a show of support. The next week, I was granted tenure. I had my job, and I had it on my terms.

Soon thereafter I was approached by an editor at *Independent School*, the professional journal for private school educators, to write an article about my experiences as an openly gay teacher.

"Why me?" I asked. "I'm a 24-year-old nobody."

"You're the only one we can find," was the response.

I wrote the article. Soon after that, I began getting calls. Many were from schools that wanted to address homophobia, and I was soon on the workshop-and-conference-presentation circuit. Suddenly, I was an expert, just because I had come out! I dutifully read all the articles written about gay issues in education in 1988 (both of them) and did my best. It seemed to be good enough, as I kept getting invited back.

After each presentation, two kinds of people would come up to me. One would be lesbian or gay teachers. Usually terrified, they often spoke in whispers, wishing they could do something about the homophobia they faced in their schools, but clearly convinced that they probably never could or would. The second type was the sympathetic straight teacher, with a gay brother or a lesbian aunt, who wanted to do something but seemed completely perplexed as to how to proceed. Frustrated, I called Kathy Henderson, a lesbian friend who taught in Andover, Massachusetts; and we came up with an idea: We would found an organization that would bring all these people together behind the single goal of ending homophobia in our schools. GLSTN was born.

One of our first problems was to gain credibility; and we decided to approach Richard Barbieri, executive director of the Association of Independent Schools in New England, to ask him to sponsor the organization as a standing committee of his association. He quickly agreed, and having his backing gave us instant respectability. We were quite clear about one basic principle: This had to be a group *anyone* could join. Sexual orientation, occupation, and type of school in which one worked were all irrelevant, we decided. All that mattered was that you saw ending homophobia in schools as a good thing. That made you eligible to join.

This principle is what keyed GLSTN's explosive growth. It wasn't as though we were the first homosexuals to think of starting a teachers' group. Numerous local groups preceded us, and the major teachers unions even had gay/lesbian caucuses. But GLSTN is unique in its focus on action and its philosophy of inclusion of people of all sexual orientations and occupations. People who came to our events knew that they would not be coming to a potluck to commiserate over the difficulty of being a gay teacher, a strategy meeting on union negotiating, or a consciousness-raising session on the evils of homophobia. What they would get was practical, hands-on advice on how to go back home and make change. We decided early on that a successful event was one that left the participant with a concrete resource. If you did not leave with something you could use, we had failed. That was our philosophy. And it worked.

One of our first problems was to gain credibility . . .

Our first conference, in 1991, drew 80 people, mainly from Massachusetts. Our fourth, in 1994, drew more than 400; and they came from more than 20 states. It became clear that there is a pent-up demand for an organization of GLSTN's nature, and interest has grown as we have established a track record of success.

By 1994 GLSTN had become known nationally as one of the key forces in the drive that made Massachusetts the first state in the nation to ban discrimination on the basis of sexual orientation in its public schools. GLSTN members developed the recommendations that formed the basis of the Massachusetts Governor's Commission on Gay and Lesbian Youth's report, *Making Schools Safe for Gay and Lesbian Youth*; GLSTN members developed the "Gay-Straight Alliance" student program, which was the key recommendation of the Commission; GLSTN was chosen to develop the faculty training component of the Massachusetts Department of Education's "Safe Schools for Gay and Lesbian Students" Program — the first program sponsored by a state government to end homophobia in schools; and GLSTN was honored for this work with a proclamation by Massachusetts Governor William Weld in 1993.

Organizing Nationally

At the same time, a consensus was growing across the country that something needed to be done about homophobia in schools. The 1989 *Report on*

Youth Suicide of the U.S. Department of Health and Human Services — which showed that gay youth are three times more likely to attempt suicide than their heterosexual peers — galvanized many who were previously unconcerned. Those individuals began to look for a resource to call on to make change. For many, GLSTN was that resource; and increasing numbers of our members were coming from outside of Massachusetts and New England.

By spring 1994 a new problem became apparent to us. While there were many interesting individuals and local efforts around the country, there was no central focus for antihomophobia work in schools. While anti-gay forces were unified and focused, pro-diversity groups were small, weak, and divided — where they even existed. Thus, at the prodding of folks from other parts of the country, we decided to try to build a new national entity — one based on local chapters that would develop programming appropriate for their communities but also linked together in a national network to increase their resources and strengths. In this way, we could respect the diversity of the challenges facing different communities but also have a way to share ideas and make sure the wheel was not being constantly re-invented.

We took the advice of Ben Franklin to delegates at the Continental Congress, who were bickering in 1775 as British forces closed in on the young nation struggling to survive: "We must all hang together or, most assuredly, we will all hang separately."

Since then, GLSTN's growth has been phenomenal. Local chapters have been or are being formed in more than 20 areas, including Atlanta, Boston, Chicago, Cincinnati, Cleveland, Colorado, Columbus, Connecticut, Dallas, D.C., Detroit, Indianapolis, Los Angeles, New Hampshire, New Mexico, New York, Philadelphia, Portland (Maine), Portland (Oregon), St. Louis, Tampa, and Washington State. In 1994-95, GLSTN successfully staged regional conferences in Los Angeles, Louisville, Philadelphia, and Santa Fe, drawing more than 900 people in addition to the 500 who attended GLSTN's 1995 national conference in Boston.

GLSTN helped local groups introduce legislation to protect the rights of gay and lesbian youth into the state legislatures of California and Connecticut during the 1995 legislative session. And GLSTN assisted many local groups doing similar work at the school board level. Virtually overnight, a national network of groups united behind the idea of ending homophobia.

> *GLSTN's growth has been phenomenal.*

Important Lessons

The success of this effort was based on three key factors. The lessons for those seeking to organize effective work to end homophobia in schools are clear:

1. Frame the issue the right way. In order to understand this lesson, we first must understand some history. Throughout history, minorities have been stereotyped as preying on children. This stereotype is used in an effort to frighten the majority into opposing equality for all. In the late 19th century, Russian Jews were accused of killing Christian children in order to use their blood in the Passover Seder, a myth used to justify pogroms. In the American South of the early 20th century, black men were accused of molesting white girls, which justified the lynching of African-American males. Today gay men and lesbians are routinely portrayed as pedophiles in an effort to justify discrimination, even though a 1993 *Pediatrics* study found that a child is 100 times more likely to be molested by a heterosexual man than by a gay one.

Such attacks are common in gay history. There is a direct line connecting Anita Bryant's "Save our Children" campaign of the late 1970s to the campaign slogan, "Protect Our Children," used in the Oregon anti-gay referendum vote of 1994. This pattern tells us to expect attacks along these lines if we decide to do anti-homophobia work in schools.

Ironically, these attacks are successful because they appeal to a good impulse. The number-one concern of every parent is, as it should be, their child's safety. Such attacks are designed to convince parents that we are a threat to their children's safety because, if they can be convinced of this, they will oppose any protections for such a dangerous group. If the Radical Right can succeed in portraying gays as preying on children, there is no way inclusive programming can be implemented in a school. The parents simply won't stand for it.

Recognizing this, we decided that we had to define the agenda for ourselves. We have seen that our opponents have no compunction about distorting the content and intent of previous efforts to create change: witness their photocopying of pornography that was then distributed as the supposed "lesson plans" of the ill-fated "Rainbow Curriculum" in New York, a Nixonian "dirty trick" that was critical in the defeat of what was actually an innocuous program.

In Massachusetts, the effective reframing of this issue was the key to our success. We immediately seized on the opponent's calling card — safety — and turned it to our favor by showing how homophobia represents a threat to students' safety, as it creates a climate in which violence, name-calling, health problems, and suicide are common. Titling our report, "Making Schools Safe for Gay and Lesbian Youth," we automatically threw our opponents onto the defensive and stole their best line of attack. This framing short-circuited their arguments and left them back-pedaling from the outset.

When we decided to take GLSTN national, we knew that we once again had to be very clear in what we were about, or else we would find our words and intents distorted and twisted by people who sought to portray us as something we were not. We spent a great deal of time working on developing a clear mission statement to avoid such distortion. The following was adopted by our board in August 1994:

> The Gay, Lesbian, and Straight Teachers Network strives to assure that each member of every school community is valued and respected, regardless of sexual orientation. We believe that such an atmosphere engenders a positive sense of self, which is the basis of educational achievement and personal growth. Since homophobia and heterosexism undermine a healthy school climate, we work to educate teachers, students, and the public at large about the damaging effects these forces have on youth and adults alike. We recognize that forces such as racism and sexism have similarly adverse impacts on communities, and we support schools in seeking to redress all such inequities. GLSTN seeks to develop school climates where difference is valued for the positive contribution it makes in creating a more vibrant and diverse community. We welcome as members anyone who is committed to seeing this philosophy realized in K-12 schools.

In reaching out to unfamiliar people, we felt it was critical to frame our mission in positive terms linked to values we all share. After all, who can be against "valuing and respecting" everyone? Who can oppose "healthy school climates"? Who thinks a "positive sense of self" is a bad thing? Who decries "educational achievement"? Framing our values in terms that could appeal to everyone is vital for winning acceptance, rather than creating defensiveness. Too often advocates of equality for gay people are put in the position of saying "No" ("No on 9") or being *against* something (homophobia, heterosexism, bad hair, whatever). We felt it was critical, instead, to be *for* something. It is easier to work for something positive than against something negative, and this forward-looking approach has been one that many observers have cited as one of the GLSTN's best features.

2. Organize across existing divisions. Just as the values espoused must be universal in nature, so must the approach taken in gaining new members. If we are truly about equality for all, we must include all people. This has been an underlying premise of GLSTN's work from the beginning, and another feature that many new members have cited as one of the organization's most attractive.

This feature also was part of a strategic decision made when we chose to "go national" in the spring of 1994. Straight people had always been welcomed in GLSTN — even when we used our original name, "The Gay and Lesbian School Teachers Network." However, some of our active straight members pointed out that their friends did not feel comfortable in coming to GLSTN, as they perceived it as a "gay only" group. "Gay-only" had never been our approach: the "Gay-Straight Alliance," open to any student, had been one of our most successful programs, and we felt it was important that such a philosophy pervade the organization. As a result, we decided to keep the old acronym, but do a little switch: in 1994, GLSTN became "The Gay, Lesbian, and *Straight* Teachers Network."

The response to this change was electric. Straight allies felt a new sense of inclusion; and gay, lesbian, and bisexual folks felt a new sense of validation from the influx of straight people who saw this as their fight, too. In addition to adding numbers, the shift involved an important psychic shift as well. GLSTN was not about advancing a "gay agenda" or setting up support groups. Instead, we became identified as a group about equality and justice, which are values that are held not only by gay people but also by most Americans. We wanted to model in GLSTN what we wanted to see in society at large — gay and straight people working together. If gay and straight people in GLSTN were truly "together, for a change" (our new slogan), then per-

We wanted to model in GLSTN what we wanted to see in society at large — gay and straight people working together.

257

haps it would be possible to see this happen in our classrooms and school corridors as well.

3. Put a human face on the argument. Homophobia is a form of defamation that is fueled by the ability of anti-gay people to depict gays as a frightening "others." If gays are faceless, it is that much easier for hate-mongers to put a negative spin on our intentions and character. Knowing this, we decided that a central strategy for GLSTN would be to put a human face on the "homosexual monster" (as I was once called by an administrator of my college). We needed to make real for the community the pain that gay people endure in schools, and we set about doing that by confronting resistant or ignorant folks with real stories so that they would "get it." We knew that, faced with real-life stories of youth who had suffered from homophobia, it would be hard for people to deny the need to take action. We wanted other school people, such as school board members, to have an actual kid in mind when they had to cast votes on our proposals. And we knew that this strategy had worked in the past, for example, when we brought the gay student rights bill to the Massachusetts senate in 1993, where we won the final vote 33-7. Virtually the same senate had passed the gay civil rights law by a slim four-vote margin only three years earlier. If we could tell a story, we could win a heart — and a mind would follow.

Therefore, from the beginning, we emphasized such stories in our work. Throughout our literature we sprinkled quotes from our students, words that drove home the message that the inaction of schools harmed them. Examples included:

> "I was pushed, kicked, thrown against lockers, and — worst of all— spit upon, like some vile piece of trash." 16-year-old gay boy

> "I hear homophobic comments all the time in my classes. Sometimes I think teachers don't hear what goes on in their classrooms. I want teachers to remember that I can't block out the homophobia. I hear it even when I don't want to listen. I hear it every day that I am in this school. And it hurts a lot." 16-year-old lesbian

> "Straight kids have all kinds of people they can talk to at the high school for advice and help in their personal lives. Lesbians and gays don't. We can't go to teachers because you don't know how they're going to react. And we can't go to friends for the same reason." 16-year-old lesbian

Homophobia is un-American. . . . I can't imagine a better lesson for any educator — gay, lesbian, or straight — to teach.

"I was very different from other students and they picked up on it. Immediately the words 'faggot' and 'queer' were used to describe me. Freshman year of high school was hard enough; but with the big seniors pushing you around because the rumor is you're the faggot, it's ten times worse. I knew I was gay. But who could I talk to? I was spit upon, pushed, and ridiculed. My school life was hell. I decided to leave school because I couldn't handle it. " 17-year-old gay boy

"I go to school every day, afraid of violence, feeling that I can't be honest, that I have no right to be proud, that I am a second-class citizen." 17-year-old lesbian

Faced with these testimonies, educators find it hard to say that our work isn't important. Opponents were similarly chagrined. Such testimony automatically put them on the defensive because, in order to attack our program, they would have to attack people who already had been victimized once, which would cast them as bullies and make it hard to emerge looking good. No one likes somebody who beats up on a kid. Even the most retrograde opponents found themselves having to begin their rebuttals by saying, "Now, of course, I think what happened to these kids was awful. . . ," which allowed us to ask immediately, "Then why aren't you willing to do something to help?" They often were at a loss for an answer.

An unanticipated benefit for us was the empowerment brought to the youth themselves by the opportunity to tell their stories. Initially I worried about "exposing" the youth by asking them to speak out publicly, but they just seemed to get stronger and stronger, drawing strength from the chance to finally speak out about the obstacles they faced. They often became the fiercest advocates, willing to go far beyond their teachers in their determination to confront recalcitrant administrators and politicians. Far from having to "protect" them, we often found ourselves thinking we'd better protect the administrators that the kids we were after!

Inspired by these successes, in the fall of 1995 we decided to initiate our most ambitious program. Called the "Back-to-School Campaign," this is a national effort to get every gay adult to write to a teacher at their old school, first, to make sure their former teachers know what it was like for one gay youth they know and, second, to demand to know what is being done for today's gay kids. The goal is similarly two-fold: first, to involve gay people with the schools again, because the majority of gay adults do not have children and thus have little cause to interact directly with the education system; and second, to make sure that teachers know that homophobia is a problem in their classes, even if they do not yet know who their gay students are. We hope to make sure that every educator in America has a human face in mind when it comes time to address homophobia. Teachers are good people; they've chosen the profession because they care about kids. The thrust of our work is to remind them that, if they really do care about kids, then they need to address homophobia because it hurts kids. It's that simple.

Conclusion

One always feels nervous touting one's success before the "fat lady sings" (if you will pardon the politically incorrect idiom). The opponents of equality for gay people are well-funded and determined and willing to stoop to virtually anything to win. Our program calls on people to overcome their stereotypes, to leave behind old ways of thinking, and to embrace a new way of relating — one that is, in the end, healthier, happier, and more in line with American values of justice, equality, and fairness than is the status quo. But the new way of relating also is new, frightening (for some), and a departure from accepted ways of thinking.

The jury is still out on whether people will take the leap of faith necessary to embrace our work. Some think we may not succeed. I do not share that view. I do know that it may not be easy. After all, it took our nation 100 years to get the idea that slavery was inconsistent with our most fundamental values and even longer to understand that denying suffrage to women violated those same values. But we did *eventually* get it, and I think we are on the verge of doing the same on equality for gay people.

Why am I confident? Because I went to public schools in this country, schools where each day I pledged allegiance to a flag that, I was taught, stood for "liberty and justice for all." Homophobia is un-American; it violates the pledge we've all said since we were little kids in elementary school. Full equality for gay and lesbian individuals may be a new idea, but it's one we're starting to learn. I can't imagine a better lesson for any educator — gay, lesbian, or straight — to teach.

Preventing Gay Teen Suicide

by Frances Snowder

Gay* youth are most at risk of suicide during the critical adolescent years when they are attempting to explore their own identities and to form adult emotional relationships. This is a time when they need the most support from family, peers, and others. Unfortunately, many gay youth do not find such support in their homes or schools.

Gay teens represent a significant percentage of the adolescents who commit or attempt suicide. Approximately 500,000 adolescents attempt suicide every year (Hicks 1990, p. 9). Recent reports confirm that more than 5,000 succeed, and at least 30% of completed suicides (or some 1,500 each year) are gay youth. In addition, gay youth are two to six times more likely to attempt suicide than heterosexual youth (Remafedi 1994, p. 17).

Many homeless children are on the streets because they have run away or been cast out of their homes because of conflicts over their sexual orientation. Youth in schools who remain anonymous and silent often have been frightened into emotional isolation by the prevalent homophobic environment. They often choose not to confide in authority figures, such as teachers and counselors, whom they fear will diminish or disregard their feelings; expose them to embarrassment, ridicule, or harassment; or try to "cure" them.

Unfortunately, the concerns of gay teens are not adequately addressed in the literature for teachers, school administrators, health providers, and guid-

---

*In the context of this essay, "gay" is an inclusive term comprising all sexual minorities: homosexual males, lesbians, and bisexual and transsexual individuals.

ance counselors. In fact, until recent years, the numerous studies done on adolescents and suicide failed even to mention gay youth.

Research on Gay Teen Suicide

. . . a major problem with researching matters pertaining to teen sexual orientation is the lack of reliable information.

Although pioneering research on gay teen suicide was done by physicians Ronald F.C. Kourany (1987) and Gary Remafedi as early as the mid-1980s, the national alert in the United States was not sounded until 1989 by Paul Gibson's ground-breaking article, "Gay Male and Lesbian Youth Suicide" in *Report of the Secretary's Task Force on Youth Suicide,* published by the U.S. Department of Health and Human Services. This controversial report to the Bush Administration first stated that gay teens account for 30% of all youth suicides.

Unfortunately, questions about the reliability of the report's statistics superseded any positive political action. However, the 30% statistic holds fast in a recently published book, *Death by Denial: Studies of Suicide in Gay and Lesbian Teenagers,* edited by Gary Remafedi (1994). An anthology of the major research on the subject, Remafedi's book republishes his own 1991 article (cited below) along with Kourany's 1987 article, "Suicide Among Homosexual Adolescents," and the Gibson report. Though far from comprehensive, this book, which contains only four other major research articles and the text of the state legislation passed by the Governor's Commission on Gay and Lesbian Youth in Massachusetts, is regarded as the most authoritative text on the subject to date.

Of the included studies, most deal exclusively with gay and bisexual males. Those studies that include all of the various sexual minorities as a total group tend to slight the issues for lesbians and transsexual youth and omit the effects of various gender proscriptions in racial and ethnic minority cultures. The fact that most of the articles now are several years old also indicates that sexual minority suicide is a subject that requires much more serious scholarly attention.

However, a major problem with researching matters pertaining to teen sexual orientation is the lack of reliable information. It is virtually impossible at this time to get fully truthful and accurate data on homosexuality, because the subject is so stigmatized and access to the underage teen population is difficult to obtain. Most statistics on teen sexual orientation are based on surveys that ask respondents to self-report.

In addition to a lack of dependable research data on gay teens in general, other factors obstruct the collection of data on gay teen suicide. Data on suicide is collected in different ways from various states and even from counties within states. Cultural taboos against suicide and homosexuality also tend to result in the under-reporting of gay suicides. Families may conceal information, for example, reporting suicides as accidents.

Cultural norms also may obscure teen suicide issues. For example, researcher Joyce Hunter quotes H.F. Myers, who reports, "Black gay youths may be more inclined to provoke others to kill them rather than to commit suicide; such victim-precipitated homicide may mask the frequency of suicide in this group" (Hunter 1994, p. 104).

Known Risk Factors

Certainly, further research is necessary to help educators fully understand these matters, but today's teachers and administrators can deal with what already is known. For example, in "Risk Factors for Attempted Suicide in Gay and Bisexual Youth," Remafedi, Farrow, and Deisher (1991) contend that most gay youth suicides are committed by teens dealing *for the first time* with issues of sexual orientation and identity. In this study of attempted suicide survivors who subsequently identified themselves as gay, the authors reported that "almost one-third of subjects made their first suicide attempt in the same year that they identified themselves as bisexual or homosexual. Overall, three-fourths of all first attempts temporally followed self-labeling" (p. 871).

Although declassified as a psychopathologic illness in 1973 by the American Psychiatric Association, homosexuality often is still treated as an abnormality in many clinical settings. This situation led the American Medical Association to repudiate "reparative" therapy in 1994, calling instead for a "non-judgmental recognition of sexual orientation" by physicians (Brinkley 1994, p. 1). For school people, this evolving attitude should signal an awareness that, unlike other troubled adolescents who are at-risk for suicide, gay teens may be psychologically healthy; but gay teens must cope with a gay-hostile environment that, if internalized, can be destructive to self-esteem — and survival.

Hostility may be physical as well as psychological. Fear and hatred of gay and lesbian youth are acted out in name-calling and physical abuse. Verbal and physical abuse most often occur at home and in school, both places where most teenagers might expect to be protected and to feel safe. In a study conducted by the National Gay and Lesbian Task Force, 45% of the gay men and 20% of the lesbians surveyed had been victims of verbal and physical assaults in secondary school because of their sexual orientation (Center for Population Options 1992).

Another study of 500 New York City youths served by a gay youth services agency revealed that 46% of those who had experienced a violent physical attack reported that the assault was gay-related. Of those who had experienced violence in their homes, 61% reported the abuse as gay-related (Center for Population Options 1992).

In 1993 the Massachusetts Governor's Commission on Gay and Lesbian Youth reported a study that surveyed 218 adolescents at seven community-based gay and lesbian youth groups and eight school-based gay/straight alliances across Massachusetts (Remafedi 1994, pp. 199-200). The responses to four of the 33 survey questions are noteworthy. (Category totals may not equal 100% because of rounding.)

"How would most students in your high school react to finding out a student they knew was lesbian, gay, or bisexual?"

Negative	60%
Neutral	21%
Mixed	13%
Positive	5%

"How would the parents of most of your friends react to finding out that their child was lesbian, gay, or bisexual?"

Negative	60%
Neutral	17%
Positive	17%
Mixed	7%

"Have you ever heard teachers in your high school make anti-lesbian or anti-gay remarks?"

Yes	53%
No	47%

"How often do you hear anti-gay or anti-lesbian remarks made at your high school?"

Sometimes	51%
Often	43%
Never	6%

Ritch C. Savin-Williams' research on verbal and physical abuse as stressors in the lives of lesbians, gay males, and bisexual youths associates substance abuse, promiscuity, alcoholism, running away, and delinquency among gay teens with crises over sexual orientation (1994). And, as would be expected, Savin-Williams found a strong correlation between such self-destructive behavior patterns and suicide attempts.

To the detriment of many gay teens, their peers, parents, teachers, and counselors have failed to recognize the connections between homophobia and the suicide risks for gay youth. Diane Allensworth, speaking as associate executive director for programs for the American School Health Association, stated that a recent survey of its members who are school nurses and health teachers revealed that "homosexuality was the number one topic they weren't equipped to discuss" (Buss 1993, p. 71).

Similarly, a study of 289 secondary school counselors published in the December 1991 *Journal of School Health* reported that "17% thought there were no gay students in their school and 20% thought they would not be competent counseling gay students" (Center for Population Options 1992).

James T. Sears, an associate professor of education at South Carolina University, has used a number psychological instruments to document the highly negative attitudes toward gays of students, teachers, prospective teachers, and guidance counselors in the schools. For example, a survey of prospective teachers and existing counselors found that "eight out of ten prospective teachers harbored negative feeling towards lesbians and gay men. One-third were classified as 'high grade homophobics.' Two-thirds of existing coun-

To the detriment of many gay teens, their peers, parents, teachers, and counselors have failed to recognize the connections between homophobia and the suicide risks for gay youth.

selors expressed negative attitudes and feelings about homosexuality and less than one-quarter have chosen to counsel homosexual students" (Harbeck 1991, pp. 29-75).

Reducing the Risks

Sexual awareness and self-knowledge and identity are part of living — and should be part of learning.

If gay youth are allowed to be themselves and the issues of gay teens are adequately addressed by teachers, guidance counselors, and health workers, many suicides can be prevented. The necessity of leading a stigmatized and sometimes double life is a heavy burden for an adult. It is even heavier for an adolescent first coming to terms with issues of identity and sexuality. Without role models, without support from friends and family, gay teenagers often are unable to complete the critical transition to adulthood. Suicide, at that low point, is considered a way out. And now a terrible new trend has been identified: purposely contracting AIDS. (Carey 1994).

How, then, can educators reduce the risks to gay youth? Following are three basic suggestions:

First, nondiscrimination policies regarding sexual orientation would aid in suicide prevention efforts in the schools. Such policies would prohibit teachers, students, and others from verbally or physically harassing gay students (or colleagues). If such policies were publicized and enforced, they would inspire trust and boost the self-esteem of gay students.

When school policies set the tone for a gay-supportive school environment and resources are available to gay students, students who are anxious or questioning about their sexual orientation will be more likely to seek the help of teachers and counselors. However, when gay students go to their teachers and counselors with their problems, those professionals need to be adequately informed about the issues and in a position to help.

Thus a second suggestion is in order: Proactive schools will need to devote time and money to staff development. Schools that adopt a proactive stance on gay youth issues also may wish to seek out openly gay educators and other professionals to lead workshops and seminars. If the limitations of regional politics prohibit such a direct approach, then school leaders, at the very least, can provide professional literature on gay issues and access for teachers and counselors to seminars and other forms of training at regional and national conferences or through university classes.

Third, schools should provide "safe" options for students to learn about their sexuality and to discuss sexual orientation issues. Many youth in distress over sexual orientation and identity do not wish to "come out of the closet" to individuals in their school, no matter how accepting the school environment is. Therefore, indirect approaches also should be developed, such as providing information brochures in the library or counseling center. Resource addresses and telephone hotline numbers can be posted on easily accessible bulletin boards. A selection of gay fiction and nonfiction books can be maintained openly in the school library. Gay-affirmative literature and services should be provided in schools so that the legitimate issues of gay youth can be discussed openly.

These efforts will help to make discussions and information about sexual issues a normal part of the learning process. Sexual awareness and self-knowledge and identity are part of living — and should be part of learning. When the subject of homosexuality is normalized by and for educators and other service providers, public opinion will change and homophobia can be reduced. Then teens, who once would have struggled to understand their sexual identity alone and in fear, will be able to find accurate information, sympathetic understanding, and simple acceptance from educators they trust and respect. Such an environment will help to maintain and enhance healthy self-esteem, and gay teens will no longer be at risk of suicide.

References

Brinkley, Sidney. "New AMA Policy a 'Landmark'." *Washington Blade* 16 (December 1994): 1.

Buss, Dale. "Homosexual Rights Go to School." *Christianity Today* 37 (17 May 1993): 70-73.

Carey, Rae, coordinator of the National Advocacy Coalition on Youth and Sexual Orientation in Washington, D.C. Personal communication. 15 November 1994.

Center for Population Options. "Lesbian, Gay and Bisexual Youth: At Risk and Underserved." Fact Sheet. Washington, D.C., September 1992.

Gibson, Paul. "Gay Male and Lesbian Youth Suicide." In *Report of the Secretary's Task Force on Youth Suicide 3: Preventions and Interventions in Youth Suicide*. Washington, D.C.: U.S Department of Health and Human Services, January 1989.

Harbeck, Karen M. *Out of the Classroom Closet: Gay and Lesbian Students, Teachers and Curricula*. Binghampton, New York: (Harrington Park Press, 1991).

Hicks, Barbara Barrett. *Youth Suicide: A Comprehensive Manual for Prevention and Intervention*. Bloomington, Ind.: National Educational Service, 1990.

Hunter, Joyce. "Violence Against Lesbian and Gay Male Youths." In *Death by Denial: Studies of Suicide in Gay and Lesbian Teenagers*, edited by Gary Remafedi. Boston: Alyson, 1994.

Kourany, Ronald F.C. "Suicide Among Homosexual Adolescents." *Journal of Homosexuality* 13, no. 4 (1987): 111-17.

Remafedi, Gary, ed. *Death by Denial: Studies of Suicide in Gay and Lesbian Teenagers*. Boston: Alyson, 1994.

Remafedi, Gary; Farrow, James; and Deisher, Robert. "Risk Factors for Attempted Suicide in Gay and Bisexual Youth." *Pediatrics* 87 (June 1991): 869-75.

Savin-Williams, Ritch C. "Verbal and Physical Abuse as Stressors in the Lives of Lesbian, Gay Male, and Bisexual Youths: Associations with School Problems, Running Away, Substance Abuse, Prostitution, and Suicide." *Journal of Consulting and Clinical Psychology* 62 (April 1994): 261-69.

Part Five
Resources

Resources

Compiled with assistance from
Lea E. Dickson

Listed in this section is a sampling of the many print, audio, and video resources available for educators, parents, and students. Likewise, only a few of the more prominent organizations are listed here. The purpose of this sampling is to offer readers several starting points from which to initiate their own information gathering. The addresses and phone numbers were current as this book went to press.

One particularly noteworthy starting point is the extensive bibliography of gay and lesbian resources of all types compiled by Tracy Phariss. That bibliography can be obtained from The Teachers' Group of Colorado and is listed in the first section below.

Bibliographies, Resource Guides, and Directories

Print Resources:

Dotson, Edisol W., ed. *Putting Out: A Publishing Resource Guide of Lesbian and Gay Writers, 1991-1992-1993 Supplement.* Available from Putting Out Books, 2215-R Market Street, #113, San Francisco, CA 94114.

Editors of Out Magazine. *The Gay and Lesbian Address Box.* May 1995. Available from Perigee Books, 200 Madison Ave., New York, NY 10016.

Hetrick-Martin Institute. *You Are Not Alone: National Lesbian, Gay, and Bisexual Youth Organization Directory, Spring 1993.* Available from Hetrick-Martin Institute, 2 Astor Place, New York, NY 10003.

Lee, Judith A.B. *An Annotated Bibliography of Gay and Lesbian Readings for Social Workers and Other Helping Professions.* East Rockaway, N.Y.: Cummings and Hathaway, 1991.

Lesbian, Gay, and Bisexual Issues in Education Network. *Resource Directory, 1994-95.* Sponsored by the Association for Supervision and Curriculum Development. Available from network coordinator Jan M Goodman, P.O. Box 27527, Oakland, CA 94602.

Phariss, Tracy. *A Bibliography: Gay and Lesbian Issues in Education.* Lakewood, Colo.: The Teachers' Group of Colorado, 1994. Available from The Teacher's Group of Colorado, P.O. Box 280346, Lakewood, CO 80228-0346.

Sex Information and Education Council of the United States (SIECUS). *Gay Male and Lesbian Sexuality and Issues, 1991.* Available from SIECUS, 130 West 42nd Street, New York, NY 10036.

Organizations:

Parents, Families, and Friends of Lesbians and Gays (PFLAG)
P.O. Box 27605
Washington, DC 20038
(202) 638-4200
Fax (202) 638-0243
E-mail: PFLAGNTL@AOL.COM
Produces suggested reading lists.

Curricula and Professional Issues

Print Resources:

American Library Association. *Censorship and Selection Issues and Answers for Schools.* Chicago, 1993.

Besner, Hilda F., and Spungin, Charlotte S. *Gay and Lesbian Students: Understanding Their Needs.* Bristol, Pa.: Taylor & Francis, 1995.

Blumenfeld, Warren J., ed. *Homophobia: How We All Pay the Price.* Boston: Beacon, 1992.

Epstein, Debbie, ed. *Challenging Lesbian and Gay Inequalities in Education.* Bristol, Pa.: Open University Press, 1994.

Gay and Lesbian Alliance Against Defamation/San Francisco Bay Area. *Homophobia: Discrimination Based on Sexual Orientation.* 1990. Available from the alliance, 1360 Mission Street, Suite 200, San Francisco, CA 94103. In the Los Angeles area: GLAAD, P.O. Box 931763, Hollywood, CA 90093. (213) 463-3632.

Gayellow Pages™ The National Edition #20. New York: Renaissance House, 1994. (P.O. Box 533, Village Station, New York, NY 10014-0533.

Harbeck, Karen M. *Coming Out of the Classroom Closet: Gay and Lesbian Students, Teachers, and Curriculum.* Binghamton, N.Y.: Harrington Park Press, 1992.

Jennings, Kevin, ed. *Becoming Visible: A Reader in Gay and Lesbian History for High School and College Students.* Boston: Alyson, 1994.

Jennings, Kevin, ed. *One Teacher in Ten: Gay and Lesbian Educators Tell Their Stories.* Boston: Alyson, 1994.

Khayatt, Madiha Didi. *Lesbian Teachers: An Invisible Presence.* Albany: State University of New York Press, 1992.

McConnell-Celi, Sue, ed. *Twenty-First Century Vision: Lesbians and Gays in Education, Bridging the Gap.* Red Bank, N.J.: Lavender Crystal, 1992.

McNaught, Brian. *Gay Issues in the Workplace.* New York: St. Martin's, 1993.

Sears, James T. *Sexuality and the Curriculum.* New York: Teachers College Press, 1992.

Unks, Gerald, ed. *The Gay Teen: Educational Practice and Theory for Lesbian, Gay, and Bisexual Adolescents.* New York: Routledge, 1995.

Walling, Donovan R. *Gay Teens at Risk.* Fastback 357. Bloomington, Ind.: Phi Delta Kappa Educational Foundation, 1993.

Woog, Dan. *School's Out: The Impact of Gay and Lesbian Issues on America's Schools.* Boston: Alyson, 1995.

Organizations:

Bay Area Network of Gay and Lesbian Educators (BANGLE)
P.O. Box 460545
San Francisco, CA 94146
(415) 648-8488

Provides professional development and support services through five chapters in the San Francisco area. It is not affiliated with GLSTN.

Campaign to End Homophobia
Box 819
Cambridge, MA 02130
(617) 868-8280

Produces teaching materials. Example: *Guide to Leading Introductory Workshops on Homophobia.*

Gay and Lesbian High School Curriculum and Staff Development Project
Arthur Lipkin, Research Associate
Harvard Graduate School of Education
210 Longfellow Hall
Cambridge, MA 02138
(617) 547-2197

Produces curriculum materials. Example: *The Stonewall Riots.*

Gay, Lesbian, and Straight Teachers Network (GLSTN)
Kevin Jennings, Executive Director
122 West 26th Street, Suite 1100
New York, NY 10001
(212) 727-0135
Fax (212) 727-0254
E-mail: GLSTN@glstn.org

Publishes newsletters, sponsors educator retreats, and conducts chapter leadership training. GLSTN, founded in 1990, is building a nationwide network. Audio tapes of the 23 sessions at the GLSTN 4th Annual Conference are available from Cambridge Transcriptions, 675 Massachusetts Avenue, Cambridge, MA 02139. (617) 547-0200.

Hetrick-Martin Institute
2 Astor Place
New York, NY 10003
(212) 674-2400
TTY (212) 674-8695
Fax (212) 674-8650

Social service, education, and advocacy agency for gay, lesbian, and bisexual and homeless and runaway youth. Hetrick-Martin provides individual, group, and family counseling; training; and referrals to medical and legal services. The institute also operates the alternative Harvey Milk

School and Project First Step for homeless youth and co-sponsors the National Advocacy Coalition on Youth and Sexual Orientation.

LTN
P.O. Box 301
East Lansing, MI 48826
Nationwide and international lesbian teachers network.

National Advocacy Coalition on Youth and Sexual Orientation
Rea Carey, Coordinator
1704 Lamont St., NW
Washington, DC 20010
(202) 797-7943
Fax (202) 797-9722
The mission of NACYSO is to advocate for and with youth who are lesbian, gay, or bisexual or dealing with gender identity issues. It also provides action alerts for pending anti-gay education and youth issues.

Pacific Center for Human Growth
2712 Telegraph Avenue
Berkeley, CA 94705
(510) 548-8283 (office)
Switchboard: (510) 841-6224
Offers varied resources for sexual minorities, including a speakers' bureau that provides well-trained speakers for classes and staff meetings in the San Francisco Bay Area. The Pacific Center Switchboard provides information and resources about sexual orientation issues for callers from across the country. It operates daily from 10 a.m.to 10 p.m.

PROJECT 10
c/o Virginia Uribe
Fairfax High School
7850 Melrose Avenue
Los Angeles, CA 90046
(213) 651-5200 or (818) 441-3382.
PROJECT 10 is an on-campus counseling program in the Los Angeles Unified School District. Organized in 1984, the program also conducts

workshops and training sessions for administrators and staff and has developed the *Project 10 Handbook*, a resource directory for teachers, guidance counselors, parents, and school-based adolescent-care providers.

Public Education Regarding Sexual Oreintation Issues
(P.E.R.S.O.N.)
Jessea Greenman, Coordinator
586 62nd St.
Oakland, CA 94609-1245
(510) 601-8883
E-mail: http://ww80
w.outright.com/project21
    or <Jessea@uclink2.berkeley.edu>
    Formerly the Project 21 Curriculum Advocacy Project, P.E.R.S.O.N. is an informal alliance of organizations and individuals working to ensure that fair, accurate, and unbiased information is presented to America's youth regarding the nature and diversity of sexual orientation.

Parents and Families

Print Resources:

Aarons, Leroy. *Prayers for Bobby: A Mother's Coming to Terms with the Suicide of Her Gay Son.* San Francisco: Harper, 1995.

Arnup, Katherine, ed. *Lesbian Parenting: Living with Pride and Prejudice.* Charlottetown, Prince Edward Island, Canada: Gynergy Books, 1994.

Burke, Phyllis. *Family Values: A Lesbian Mother's Fight for Her Son.* New York: Random House, 1993.

Clark, Don. *Loving Someone Gay.* Berkeley, Calif.: Celestial Arts Publishing, 1990.

Corley, Rip. *Final Closet: The Gay Parents' Guide for Coming Out to Their Children.* Miami: Editech Press, 1990.

Dew, Robb Forman. *The Family Heart: The Memoir of When Our Son Came Out.* New York: Ballantine, 1995.

Green, G. Dorsey, and Clunis, D. Merilee. *The Lesbian Parenting Book: A Guide to Creating Families and Raising Children.* Seattle: Seal, 1995.

Preston, John, ed. (with Michael Lowenthal). *Friends and Lovers: Gay Men*

Write About the Families They Create. New York: Dutton, 1995.

Shyer, Marlene Fanta, and Shyer, Christopher. *Not Like Other Boys: Growing Up Gay, A Mother and Son Look Back*. Boston: Houghton Mifflin, 1995.

Sledge, Michael. *Mother and Son*. New York: Simon and Schuster, 1995.

Swallow, Jean, and Manassee, Geoff. *Making Love Visible: In Celebration of Gay and Lesbian Families*. Freedom, Calif.: Crossing, 1995.

Wardlaw, Carole. *One in Every Family: Dispelling the Myths About Lesbians and Gay Men*. Greenwood, S.C.: Attic, 1995.

Video Resources:

Families Come Out. (1992) Available with resource guide from 21st Century News, P.O. Box 42286, Tucson, AZ 85733. (602) 327-9555.

Organizations:

Parents, Families, and Friends of Lesbians and Gays (PFLAG)
P.O. Box 27605
Washington, DC 20038
(202) 638-4200
Fax (202) 638-0243
E-mail: PFLAGNTL@AOL.COM

Local chapters can be found across the United States. Produces publications and audio tapes.

Children of Lesbians and Gays Everywhere (COLAGE)
3023 North Clark
Box 121
Chicago, IL 60657
(312) 583-8029
Fax (312) 783-6204
In Canada:
P.O. Box 187 Stn F
Toronto, Ontario M4Y 2L5
Publishes *Just for Us*.

Periodicals

Empathy
James Sears, Editor
P.O. Box 5085
Columbia, SC 29250

Journal of Homosexuality
Haworth Press
10 Alice Street
Binghamton, NY 13904-1580

MultiCultural Education Magazine
Caddo Gap Press
3145 Geary Boulevard, #275
San Francisco, CA 94118

Speaking Out: A Forum for Sexual Minority Issues in the Boarding School Community
Al Chase, Editor
2300 Market Street, #6
San Francisco, CA 94114

Teaching Tolerance
400 Washington Avenue
Montgomery, AL 36104
YOUTH Magazine
P.O. Box 34215
Washington, DC 20005

Youth Groups

Connecticut Gay Youth Groups
Robin Passariello, Program Organizer
340 Twin Lakes Road
North Branford, CT 06471
(203) 483-9651

Horizons Youth Group
Horizons Community Services
961 West Montana
Chicago, IL 60614
(312) 929-HELP (929-4357)

IYG
P.O. Box 20716
Indianapolis, IN 46220
(317) 541-8726
Fax (317) 545-8794
Hotline: 1-800-347-TEEN (347-8336) voice/TTY
Peer-facilitated hotline for gay, lesbian, and bisexual youth operates
Thursday, Friday, Saturday, and Sunday evenings, 7:00 p.m. to 11:45 p.m.

Lambda Youth Network
P.O. Box 7911
Culver City, CA 90233
(310) 821-1139

Youth Issues

Print Resources:

Due, Linnea. *Joining the Tribe: Growing Up Gay and Lesbian in the 1990s.*
    Landover Hills, Md.: Anchor, 1995.
Grima, Tony, ed. *Not the Only One.* Boston: Alyson, 1995.
Heron, Ann, ed. *One Teenager in Ten.* Boston: Alyson, 1986.
Heron, Ann, ed. *Two Teenagers in Twenty.* Boston: Alyson, 1994.
Kuklin, Susan, ed. *Speaking Out: Teenagers Take on Race, Sex, and Identity.*
    New York: Putnam and Grosset Group, 1993.
Rench, Janice E. *Understanding Sexual Identity: A Book for Gay Teens and
    Their Friends.* Minneapolis: Lerner, 1990.
Rhoads, Robert A. *Coming Out in College.* Westport, Conn.: Bergin &
    Garvey, 1994.
Romesburg, Don, ed. *Young, Gay, and Proud!* 4th ed. Boston: Alyson, 1995.

Sherrill, Jan-Mitchell, and Hardesty, Craig A. *The Gay, Lesbian, and Bisexual Students' Guide to Colleges, Universities, and Graduate Schools.* New York: New York University Press, 1994.

Shyer, Marlene Fanta, and Shyer, Christopher. *Not Like Other Boys: Growing Up Gay, A Mother and Son Look Back.* Boston: Houghton Mifflin, 1995.

Video Resources:

From a Secret Place. (1993) Developed by Karen Heller and Bill Domonokos. Available from Fanlight Productions, 47 Halifax Street, Boston, MA 02130. 1-800-937-4113.

Gay Youth. (1992) Available from Filmmakers Library, 124 East 40th Street, #901, New York, NY 10025. (212) 808-4980.

Hate, Homophobia and Schools. (September 1995) Available from NEWIST/ CESA 7, IS 1040, University of Wisconsin-Green Bay, Green Bay, WI 54311. (414) 465-2599 or 1-800-633-7445.

School's Out: Lesbian and Gay Youth. (1993) Directed by Ron Spalding. Available from Cinema Guild, 1697 Broadway, Suite 506, New York, NY 10019-5904. (212) 246-5522. Fax (212) 246-5525

Sticks, Stones and Stereotypes. (ND) Available with teacher's guide from Equity Institute, 6400 Hollis Street, Suite 15, Emeryville, CA 94608. Phone: (510) 658-4577. Fax (510) 658-5184.

Teens Speak Out. (1993) Available with guide from 21st Century News, Inc., P.O. Box 42286, Tucson, AZ 85733. (602) 327-9555.

About the Authors

JOHN D. ANDERSON teaches high school Latin and English in Stratford, Connecticut. He also leads workshops on sensitivity in language with regard to homosexuality for graduate students and writes a newspaper column on gay and lesbian issues for the *New Haven Register*.

DAVID TIMOTHY AVELINE received an M.A. in sociology from Concordia University, Montrél, Québec, in 1991. He is now a Ph.D. candidate in the Indiana University Department of Sociology and teaches courses in human sexuality.

IAN BARNARD teaches in the Department of English and Comparative Literature and the Department of Rhetoric and Writing Studies at San Diego State University in California.

KATHRYN BROWN works with Health and Wellness at Indiana University in Bloomington. She is active in a number of community organizations and often coordinates speaker panels on gay, lesbian, and bisexual issues.

LEA E. DICKSON is a health educator. She is the co-chair of the Connecticut chapter of GLSTN and also coordinates the resource directory project of the Lesbian, Gay, and Bisexual Issues in Education network of the Association for Supervision and Curriculum Development.

JAN M. GOODMAN is a mathematics specialist at the University of California, Berkeley. She previously was an elementary school administrator in the Newark Unified School District. She also is the facilitator of the member-initiated network on Lesbian, Gay, and Bisexual Issues in Education for the Association for Supervision and Curriculum Development.

HENRY GONSHAK is an associate professor of English at Montana Tech in Butte. He has written a number of essays about his experiences in introducing gay studies to his institution.

CHRISTOPHER T. GONZALEZ, in 1987, founded the Indianapolis-based IYG, a model support organization for gay, lesbian, and bisexual youth under age 21. He died on 5 May 1994 at the age of 30 from complications of AIDS.

JILL GOVER has worked with adolescents and their families as an educator, counselor, and clinical psychologist for the past 20 years. Currently, she supervises drug and alcohol intervention and treatment programs for the Vallejo City Unified School District in California. Her most recent book is *Helping Kids from Alcoholic Families* (Minneapolis: Johnson Institute, 1992).

VICKY GREENBAUM has taught in public and private schools, including Phillips Academy (Andover) and Northfield Mt. Hermon School in Massachusetts. Currently she directs the Writing Program and conducts the chamber orchestra at Menlo School in Atherton, California.

KEVIN JENNINGS is executive director of the Gay, Lesbian, and Straight Teachers Network (GLSTN). A former history teacher, Jennings is the editor of *Becoming Visible: A Reader in Gay and Lesbian History for High School and College Students* and *One Teacher in Ten: Gay and Lesbian Educators Tell Their Stories*, both published by Alyson.

LYNN JOHNSTON is a Canadian cartoonist. For more than 15 years, her syndicated "For Better or For Worse" comic strip has been appearing in newspapers across the United States and Canada. The daily strip about the Patterson family is funny and poignant and often draws on universal truths to entertain and educate.

RITA M. KISSEN is a teacher educator at the University of Southern Maine in Gorham and founding member of the Portland, Maine, chapter of PFLAG. Her recent research forms the basis of her new book, *The Last Closet: The*

Real Lives of Lesbian and Gay Teachers, published by Heinemann in May 1996.

SHULAMIT KLEINERMAN was a student at Northfield Mt. Hermon School in Northfield, Massachusetts, when she wrote her essay, "Old Enough to Know." She now is at the University of California-Berkeley, studying music and English.

ARTHUR LIPKIN heads the Gay and Lesbian Curriculum and Staff Development Project at the Harvard Graduate School of Education. Previously he was a public high school teacher in Massachusetts.

DAVID PHILLIPS teaches in the Department of Art History at the University of Queensland in Brisbane. He was an originator of "Gay and Lesbian Cultures," the first such course to be offered in Queensland, which is known in Australia for being a politically and socially conservative state.

TONY PRINCE is an openly gay high school teacher in Louisville, Kentucky. He also contributed a chapter to *One Teacher in Ten*, edited by Kevin Jennings, which was published by Alyson Publications in 1994.

JAMES T. SEARS is an associate professor in the Department of Educational Leadership and Policies at the University of South Carolina. His academic specialties are curriculum and sexuality. He is the author of numerous articles, essays, and scholarly papers and has edited several books, including *Growing Up Gay in the South: Race, Gender, and Journeys of the Spirit* (Haworth Press, 1991).

ALAN SINFIELD is a professor of English in Cultural and Community Studies at Sussex University in Brighton in the United Kingdom.

FRANCES SNOWDER is a researcher and writer who lives in Columbia, Maryland. She is a former high school and college teacher.

JOHN WARREN STEWIG is a professor in the Department of Curriculum and Instruction at the University of Wisconsin-Milwaukee. He is a frequent writer on children's literature. His most recent book for adults is *Looking at Picture Books* (Highsmith Press, 1995). His most recent book for children is *Princess Florecita and the Iron Shoes* (Alfred A. Knopf, 1995).

VIRGINIA URIBE is the founder of Project 10, an on-campus counseling program in the Los Angeles Unified School District. Organized in 1984, the program also conducts workshops and training sessions for administrators and staff and has developed the *Project 10 Handbook*, a resource directory for teachers, guidance counselors, parents, and school-based adolescent-care providers.

DONOVAN R. WALLING is Editor of Special Publications for Phi Delta Kappa. He formerly taught English and art in the Sheboygan, Wisconsin, public schools and for the Department of Defense Dependents Schools in Germany and was an education administrator in Wisconsin and Indiana. Walling is the author of books, monographs, and articles on numerous education topics.

DAN WOOG coaches soccer at Staples High School in Westport, Connecticut, and was named the 1990 National Soccer Coaches Association of America Boys Youth Coach of the Year. He is the executive editor of Soccer America's *Youth Soccer Letter*, and his writing has appeared in various periodicals, including the *New York Times, USA Today*, and *Sports Illustrated*. Woog's latest book is *School's Out: The Impact of Gay and Lesbian Issues on America's Schools*, published by Alyson Publications in 1995.

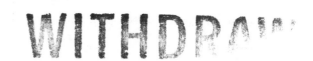